An Unexpected Detour

Kris's Story ~ *Her Difficult Journey Following a Catastrophic Stroke*

ANN COCHRAN

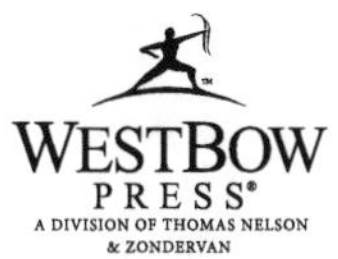

This book is a work of non-fiction. Unless otherwise noted, the author and the publisher make no explicit guarantees as to the accuracy of the information contained in this book and in some cases, names of people and places have been altered to protect their privacy.

WestBow Press books may be ordered through booksellers or by contacting:

WestBow Press
A Division of Thomas Nelson & Zondervan
1663 Liberty Drive
Bloomington, IN 47403
www.westbowpress.com
1 (866) 928-1240

ISBN: 978-1-9736-1391-6 (sc)
ISBN: 978-1-9736-1390-9 (e)

Print information available on the last page.

WestBow Press rev. date: 02/02/2018

PROLOGUE

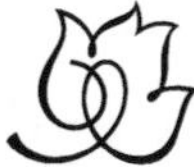

This account is being written in the hope that my recollection of things that have transpired following my stroke will be a source of information to individuals and their families who find themselves in the same situation. Some topics are not pleasant, and some seem harsh, but being thrust into the world of folks who cannot speak or act for themselves *is* harsh and difficult to comprehend. There have been several books published by individuals who suffered strokes and made fairly rapid recoveries, then went back to living their lives in pretty much the same way as they did before their episodes. Due to the severity of my own stroke, having those books read to me was informative but also caused a sense of hopelessness; I realized that I wasn't contending with the kind of stroke that could be "cured" after a short period of time. However, that knowledge also gave me a steely determination to overcome the obstacles I faced.

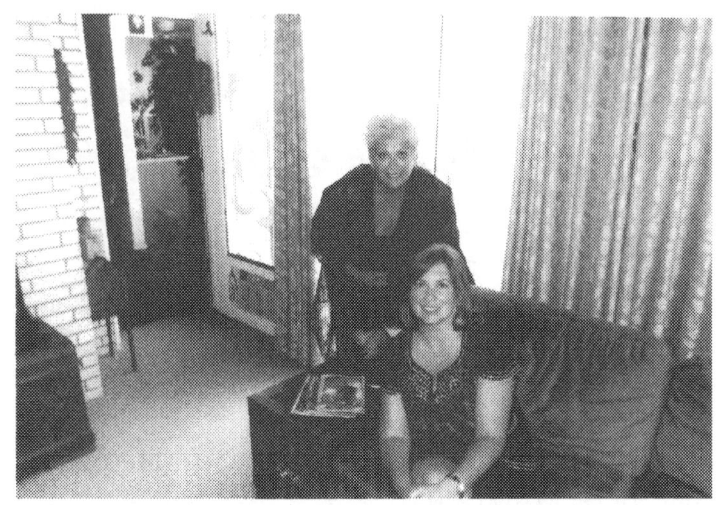

Ann Cochran, Author & Kiirstin Thomas, Her Story

My Mother, who has always been by my side and shared my sadness, frustration, fear, despondency, achievement, and finally elation, is writing this book on my behalf. I've added my input, and shared my perspective, as a former educator whose area of expertise was special education diagnostics. I now realize that the hand I've been dealt is the one that must be played; I'm the person who must make the most of the capabilities I have left following months and years of therapy. Together we have created an accounting of my extremely difficult journey from day one to where I am today. My story is by no means over, but I've arrived at a plateau where it is easy to end this narrative for the time being.

The words of my beloved grandmother, "Never give up and never ever forget who you are" guide me every day.

Kiirstin Thomas
October 2017

INTRODUCTION

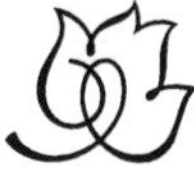

As we journey down the highways and byways of life, many times the roads we travel have already been mapped out by the direction our families have taken before us; we benefit from the guidance and experience instilled by our elders who wanted the very best for their children. Each generation hopes and dreams that their sons and daughters will be able to accomplish all that they aspire to. Mine is such a story.

My parents and grandparents wanted me to experience and try anything that came my way, from starting dance lessons at the age of two, taking gymnastics, riding scooters and mopeds, swimming fifty laps in an Olympic sized pool, or riding horses. My first memory of encouragement was from my father who said, "You can do or be anything you want once you set your mind to do it." That kind of push makes a young person think the sky is the limit, especially for a little girl who was already headstrong and willful.

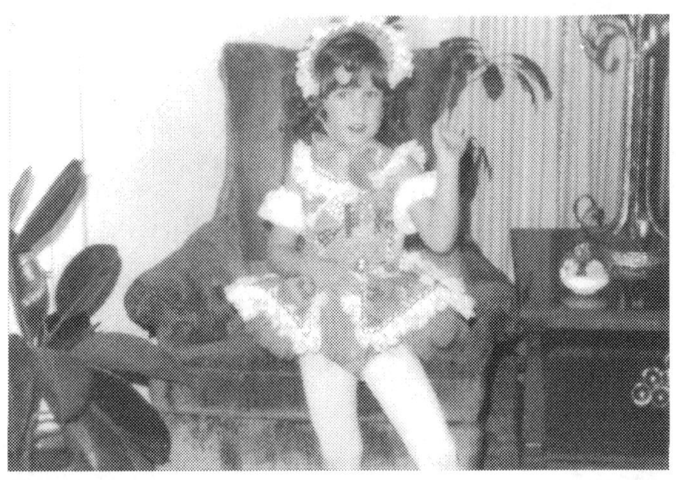

Kiirstin, age 3, "Pretty Little Maid" dance recital

I, thankfully, was afforded a good education, first attending a private girls school from kindergarten through second grade, then being enrolled in public school where it was determined that I should be placed in accelerated classes. Many times, my deportment grades did not keep pace with my scholastic ones, much to the chagrin of my parents. I was especially inventive in the second grade when I decided to record the correct spelling of words over the voice of the Nun who had taped our lesson on a recorder for the class to listen to prior to taking a test. There was no question of who the culprit was since it was my voice first slowly pronouncing the word and then spelling it out letter by letter.

About a month later, I decided the fish in the aquarium in our science class were not being fed enough, so every day when the teacher was busy with other pupils I gave them an added ration. Needless to say, the water got murky and one of the fish was floating belly up when we returned to class after a weekend. Since I was truthful ...not duplicitous enough to deny I had been meddling with the aquarium when Sister asked if anybody knew who had been putting food in the tank, I replied it was me because they looked like they were hungry. Several weeks of my allowance was spent buying new fish for the aquarium.

The coup de grace was at the end of the last semester of the second grade when the school held a book sale as a fund raiser. The book I wanted to purchase was Raggedy Ann and Andy Go to School because it came with two little dolls. I told my mother I needed $8.00 to purchase the book, and she replied that I couldn't have the money because I already had Raggedy Ann books, as well the as the dolls. Not to be denied, I decided to write a check. I took one from the back of her checkbook, filled it out completely by printing the academy's name on the payee line, filled in the numerals in the correct place, printed Eight & 00/100 on the dollar line, and finally, printed my mother's name on the signature line. The next day I gave Sister the check, picked up my purchase and brought it home on a day when my mother didn't drive the carpool; I thought I had outsmarted everybody. Four days later, the bank called Mother's office and said they had a check they would not honor due to an "irregular signature". It had cleared the teacher and the school clerk who filled out the deposit slip, but only when it got to the bank did anyone question it. You can just imagine how much trouble I was in with my Mother after that stunt ...plus, I had to return the book and dolls to the school and admit what I had done. A "check forger" at the age of seven!

I was enrolled in public school in the third grade and enjoyed the challenge of being placed in "gifted and talented" classrooms. For the most part my behavior was acceptable, but I spent more time being on restriction than many of my friends. Looking back, being sent to my room was probably the only time I wasn't arguing with my parents so I'm sure there was a "method to their madness." At one point during my last semester in junior high school, I decided I didn't want to be a nerd who made good grades, so I started listening to "heavy metal" music and not studying or turning in my schoolwork. My way of showing my classmates how "with it" I was. Grades plummeting from As to Cs and Ds for a six-week period caused me to lose all my privileges, and life wasn't nearly as cool as I thought it was going to be. Luckily for me, I was off to high school three months later and wanted to dance on a drill team where nothing less than a B was accepted, so it was back to normal and giving it my best shot every day!

My high school years were memorable; I was well behaved and made good grades due to the fact I was a member of the precision dance team. After working my way up from line girl to captain, in my junior year, I was named leader of the group.

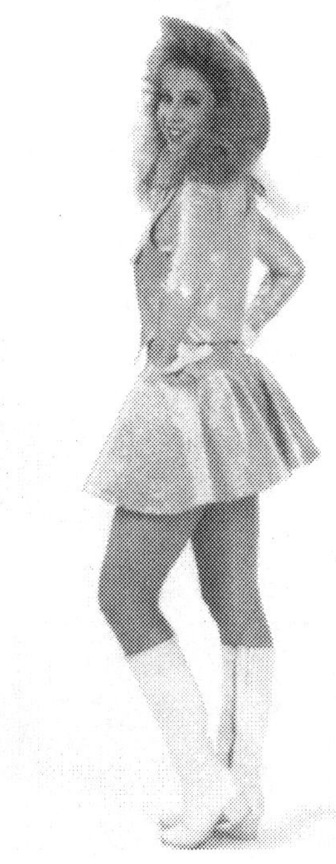

Kiirstin Cochran, Team Leader

That year my school entered our team in a national competition. Our routine was a synchronized high-kick dance performed to a rendition of "Coming to America". Our beautiful costumes were red, white and blue spangles, and when it was our turn to compete against 20 teams from across the USA, we gave an awesome spine-tingling performance that was broadcast on a national sports channel. The combination of our dance skills, enthusiasm, and patriotic music, all came together to help us win first place in the championship. Imagine our thrill and delight to bring that trophy home, especially since that was the first time any school in our little town had ever accomplished this feat – a real dream-come-true for all of us. My senior year was a whirl and plans were finalized for me to attend college 400 miles from home. What an exciting change that would be for a girl who had lived in the same house her entire life. My original field of study was pre-law, but by the end of my sophomore year, I realized practicing law would not be my choice of a career after all. Psychology had been one of the requisite courses I had taken for two years and was a subject I found very interesting, so that was my new major. I graduated two years later with a Bachelor of Science, Psychology degree. When I returned home after four years, and was ever-so-much smarter (I thought), there seemed to be few employment opportunities in that field.

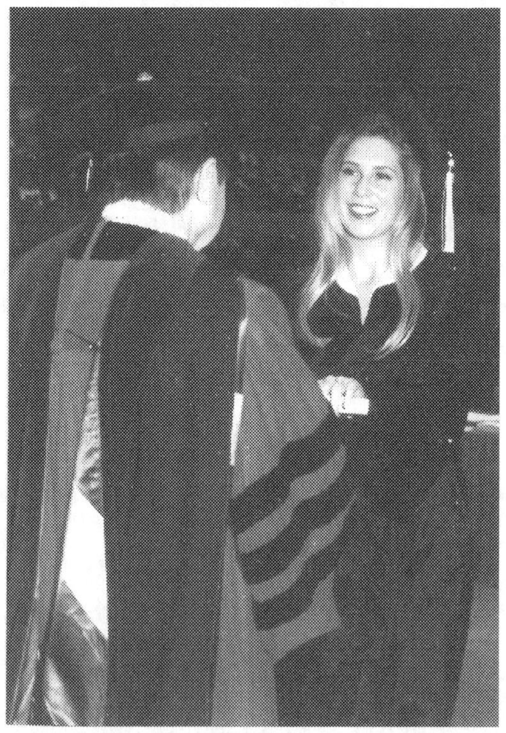

Kiirstin Cochran, B.S., Psychology

My idea of working for a progressive company in a Human Resources position, or in a large national company's EEO Department, didn't work out as I planned. Those jobs were held by women who had worked for years climbing the corporate ladder and honing their people skills. Youth and enthusiasm with zero training doesn't trump experience and life-lessons ...ever. As a matter of fact, the only job offer I got was from a government agency which would have required me to move to Washington, DC to undergo training. That wasn't something I wanted to do, so I started teaching sophomore-level students at the same high school I graduated from four and a half years earlier. This was a real wake-up call; so, at that juncture I decided to return to college and earn an alternative certification certificate to teach special education classes. As it turned out, being a Special Ed teacher was both rewarding and enjoyable. After teaching students from grades 1 thru 6 for several years, I decided to go for a Master's Degree in Special Education Diagnostics at a nearby university. That decision was made because, through the years, I had encountered too many students in my classrooms who had been incorrectly diagnosed. My lofty goal was to test and evaluate children with learning disabilities to help insure they were steered in the right direction commensurate with their own abilities. Being strong willed and of the opinion that I could do anything was still playing an important role in my life that served me well - until the *unthinkable happened* at age thirty-six, in the second year of my new job, when I was forced into the fight of my life as set forth hereafter in this book.

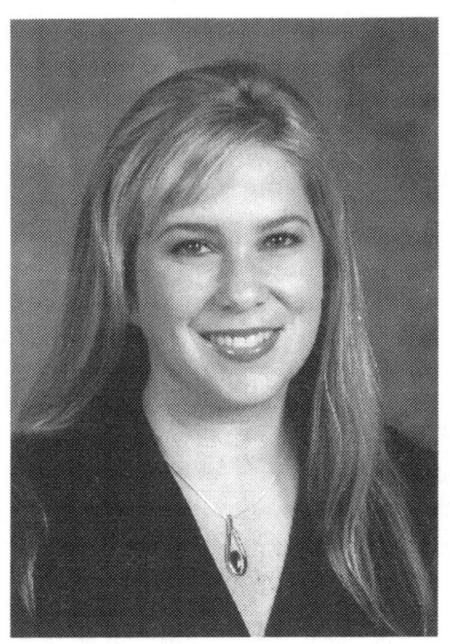

Kiirstin Thomas, M.Ed.
Educational Diagnostician

CHAPTER *One*

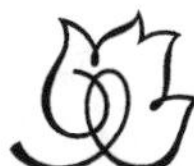

As the New Year dawned in 2009, I was full of plans. My position as a diagnostician for special education students was challenging, and each day that passed gave me a sense of accomplishment and hope for the future – especially the future of the children whose lives I touched every day. My own two-year-old son, the light of my life and reason for overwhelming joy, was just beginning to be a little person whose personality was loving and inquisitive. He learned something new each day and shared it with me when I picked him up from his daycare school e.g., "didja know that Mommy?". My career was headed down the right path, I was enjoying motherhood and each day was full of promise and love. My husband and I purchased a home the year our son was born, and it gave me such a feeling of enjoyment and fulfillment to paint and decorate and tend the yard, creating a beautiful loving environment for our family.

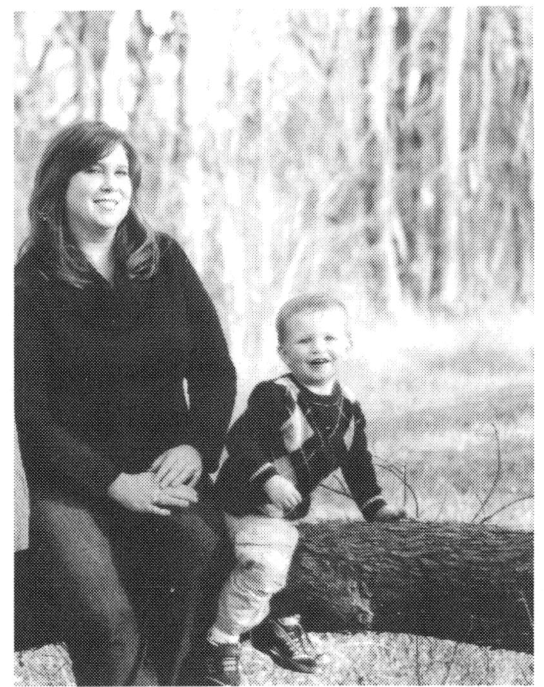

Kiirstin and Brandon, Sunday in the park

Then, March 28, 2009 was the first day of the rest of my life.

I say this because everything from the 28th until now is very different from the life I had built with such resolve. When I went to bed on the evening of March 27th, I had no way of knowing that my life would be forever changed. What happened in the early morning hours altered everything that had been part of my very being until that one moment in time.

In looking back and reconstructing the events of that evening, I remember that I had a headache and took an ansaid and a sleep aid before going to bed at 9:30 p.m. At about 2:30 a.m. I woke up and started to the kitchen for something to drink, but I was dizzy and disoriented and passed out, falling face forward on the floor. Going down, I hit my head on the bed footboard, bit my tongue and hit my hip and leg on the chest of drawers. I'm now wondering if I wasn't trying to get around to my husband Jaime's side of the bed to tell him something was wrong. When I regained consciousness, I was laying on my face/ stomach making loud unintelligible noises and calling for help, and that woke him up.

He ran around to my side of the bed and assisted me into a sitting position and kept asking me what was wrong; I didn't know anything other than coming to and finding myself on the floor. I told him to call 911. He did, and an ambulance was dispatched. I was so scared ...asked him to call my Daddy to tell him what had happened and ask him what to do. Daddy told Jaime to give me an aspirin to chew until the emergency crew got there. He suggested that I might have suffered a stroke. He held the phone for me to talk to Daddy and I managed to tell him "I love you" before we hung up. When EMS personnel got there, they opined I had suffered a stroke and called that information in to the closest hospital emergency room, so personnel would be alerted and waiting. I was then transported very quickly to that facility. As I left the house alone in the ambulance, I was extremely afraid-terrified – wondering what was going on - what in the world was happening to me? My life seemed to be going away in the blink of an eye. So very, very scared, worried about my little son Brandon. Why couldn't I move? All those thoughts tumbling through my mind ...nobody to reassure me ...all by myself ... mind just racing and utterly alone ...Oh God!

Jaime called his parents, who live approximately 25 miles away, to tell them what had happened and to ask them to meet him at the emergency room. He said he was going to wake up our son, get him dressed and then drive to the hospital as quickly as he could get there.

I was admitted to the ER; based on the symptoms EMS observed enroute to the hospital they informed the staff it was almost a certainty I had suffered a stroke. Immediately after our arrival the doctors concurred with their assessment and made a CAT scan. However, when Jaime got there they told him that the results did ***not*** show a stroke. When he and his dad came into the area where I was being observed, I was sitting up in bed and was still able to speak well enough to greet them, but I felt like I was getting worse because my head hurt, and I wasn't able to think clearly.

The Neurologist on call that morning was a renowned doctor, and was on call to cover two other hospitals. When Dr. Tim Moe arrived at the ER I had been transported to, it was almost 7:00 a.m. which was almost 4 hours after the onset of my episode. When he came in and examined me, he immediately ordered an MRI, which showed decisively that I had suffered a catastrophic stroke and there was a severe bleed in the left hemisphere of my brain. From that point on, treatment was started using his diagnosis of a dissected left carotid artery. Luckily, I don't remember any of the medical procedures they performed since it was apparently very traumatic.

Jaime called Daddy and Momma back at 8:00 a.m. to tell them what the initial diagnosis was, and to warn them that it was extremely serious. Daddy and Momma let my brother Cody and sisters Ann and Kay know before 8:30 that morning. Momma made plane reservations for she and Daddy to fly in early that evening, and Kay said she would leave home immediately and drive in to be with me that afternoon until they got there a little later.

She arrived at noon and stayed in the family waiting room, checking in on me when they would let her but mostly just sat watching and waiting. As she later told us – in an attempt to lighten the mood – that she informed everybody around me in the ER that they "better be on their A-Game because my Dad is on the way and he is very protective. Everything that should be done better be taken care of." That evening when Daddy could talk to admitting physician about what had happened to me, and asked him what he felt the prognosis was, he was very frank. Dr. Moe told him that on a severity scale of 1 to 10, my stroke was a 10. He further explained that, for whatever reason, the lining of the artery had separated, and a tear opened in the wall, which bled into the cranial cavity and caused a dissected carotid artery stroke. In my case, the tear occluded on its own before I bled out. He also explained that this type of stroke is neither hemorrhagic nor ischemic and only occurs in approximately 4 out of 100,000 cases; many times the patients are between 10 and 40 years of age, with lasting impairment always the norm. He then told my family that it would be 72-hours before they knew if my stroke would be fatal or if I would recover. That news was as bad as it possibly could have been.

The family was later informed that treatment during the first 24-hours consisted of three more MRIs to monitor what bleeding might *still* be occurring (which would have necessitated drilling a hole in my skull to relieve the pressure), insertion of a CV catheter under my right arm to the right side of my heart to monitor any kind of heart failure, and two other IVs to administer saline and steroids to help keep swelling down across the back of my brain and into the right hemisphere.

Later that evening, I was moved out of ER into a bed in the ICU telemetry unit, where all vital signs were constantly monitored to keep a watch on what was happening. It was there that I first became aware of my surroundings and realized my right arm and right leg were paralyzed. Once again, absolute terror set in ...no way to find out what was going on ...no way to talk ...the only thing I did know for sure was that *everything* was wrong. About noon the next day I was transferred to the neurology (stroke) floor, which was a Critical Care Unit, and the family was happy because they hoped that I would be getting continual personal care by qualified neurology specialists.

One of the first stroke therapists who came to evaluate my condition was the speech specialist. Visitors were asked to leave my room for their preliminary evaluation, but Daddy and Momma were standing outside the door and they heard the therapist ask questions and wait for a response. Note: Because of the bleed in my head over the prolonged period of time and the damage that caused, the speech center located in the area above my left ear was severely affected. That day – and many that followed – the only word that I could say was *"I'm."* I was trying to tell them something – anything - but the only word that came out was *"I'm."* It was absolutely devastating to not be able to tell anybody anything. It was during this examination that the speech therapist also determined that I was able to swallow, so at least that finding was good because it circumvented the necessity of a feeding tube.

In the afternoon, the next staff member who visited was a physical therapist. He manipulated my legs and arms to see if there was any feed-back regarding sensation, feeling, or movement. He cautioned Daddy and, Momma that constant care should be taken to make sure my toes weren't turned back if I slid down in the bed too far, or if sheets were cutting off circulation, because I had absolutely no feeling in my arm or leg. He also said to make sure that the skin on my arm had a pink tinge and didn't look waxy because, in the case of a stroke, skin surface and circulation were drastically impaired; it was necessary that someone gently massage my arm and leg whenever they thought about it, but at the very least every two hours. Additionally, they were warned that if it should become necessary to move me, it was imperative that my right shoulder and arm be immobilized and then moved together to keep from pulling my arm out of the socket. I couldn't really understand anything that they were saying but the scared looks on my family's faces and the tears in their eyes *said it all.*

Unfortunately, after Sunday rounds were made, Dr. Moe, was no longer involved with my treatment since he was a weekend "floater" and the hospital "staff" physicians would be taking over. Early Monday morning, a member of the neurology department staff came in and made a cursory exam, reporting that my condition appeared to be unchanged. He also noted there was no more swelling, which was a good thing since more swelling would have indicated continued bleeding and a crisis. He told Daddy and Jaime that the chief of neurology would be coming to examine me at 3:00 o'clock that afternoon; everybody started waiting patiently for the opportunity to confer to ascertain what treatment protocol would be followed. After 3:00 o'clock came and went without anyone showing up, everybody's nerves started to get raw. Fear of the unknown and perceived inactivity are real stress inducers.

The doctor from the morning shift returned at 4:00 p.m. and said that the neurologist he had referred to earlier had been detained at another hospital, but that they could expect a visit on Tuesday for sure. Even though Daddy and Momma, along with Jaime and his parents were all there early Tuesday morning, and waited patiently throughout the day for the doctor's arrival, no one came in to interface with them and answer their questions and serious concerns about me.

My day was spent being seen by speech therapists who were trying to determine if I had made any progress in being able to communicate. They had me attempt to sing the "ABC Song" and do mouth exercises. The physical therapist came in and helped me sit up; he then carefully swung my legs over to the side of the bed where he could massage my right foot, leg, and arm. He told the family that since my brain was still trying to process everything that had happened; any exertion – either mental or physical – would be extremely tiring for me. As a result of all this activity, I knew that I was seriously damaged, and that knowledge itself made me unbelievably sad and depressed; I couldn't move one side of my body and I couldn't talk. *I was begging God to let me die.* After those two therapy sessions I slept for quite a while, only rousing when a CCU staff physician and an associate of the absent head of the department came to check on me. My family's numerous questions to the nurses only garnered the rote reply that it was customary for all doctors assigned to a case to come by on a daily basis. None of them would volunteer information any further than that, so nobody knew if the inattention to my case was a normal wait-and-see policy, or if they were embarrassed about the doctor.

At this point, my mother-in-law was on her computer searching for "the best" neurology physicians in the area, while Momma was talking to my two educator friends about doctors and therapists at other hospitals. She was looking for the name of someone who would be a point of contact to assist in her effort to get me transferred to a stroke therapy facility ASAP. By the time the chief of the neurology department arrived at 4:30, on the fourth day of my hospitalization, the damage had been done insofar as my family's lack of confidence was concerned. Actually, no attempt was even made to alleviate their misgivings about implied non-essential exams or the timely attention to changes, either improving or worsening, of causative symptoms. The doctor flipped through my charts in a very casual manner, told us what everybody who had been covering had already said, then while looking at the ceiling vs. my family, explained that the planned treatment the next day would be taken care of by an associate. No one-on-one consult, no caring or feigned interest exam, just a snapping shut of the charting folder and a cool departure. That type of behavior, simply stated was, there wasn't a need to be concerned about this patient, she isn't going to make it. To say that was the straw that broke the camel's back is putting it mildly. Momma's efforts to affect my transfer to a different healthcare facility shifted into high gear. Fathers and uncles of my professional friends had been queried and consulted with and one doctor's name repeatedly came up as being the best in the field of stroke rehabilitation, Dr. Bryan McCall. Coordinating with "friends of friends" who worked alongside this doctor and his staff insured that it was going to happen at the soonest possible time.

On Wednesday, even though we were actively planning my release from the hospital and had informed personnel in the customer care office, a limited amount of therapy was continuing. The speech therapist didn't come, but sent the two student "observers" who had previously accompanied her. They attempted to help me say something using the sing-song method and the "ABC Song" to see if I could form words. I sang a few words of "Old McDonald Had a Farm" and some of the "ABC Song" which let everybody know that some of my cognition was there. One of the things that the therapists kept checking was whether I could swallow and if I could see out of both eyes. If either of those conditions were not positive, that would have indicated much more damage had occurred.

The physical therapist, who was very professional and caring, came back again and said he was going to swing my legs off the bed; he then told me he wanted me to try to stand on my left leg and balance for a moment before he helped me pivot and sit down in a wheelchair. Of course, he was holding me up but was encouraged that I could accomplish that much. He massaged my legs again and informed me he was going to lift me up out of the wheelchair and help me pivot back onto the side of the bed; he told me he knew I couldn't support myself but to go ahead and try so he could see how much strength and balance I actually had. After he helped me back in bed and comfortably propped up, he told Daddy and Momma that I had remarkable core strength and good balance, and was happy that I was able to perform this physical exercise even though it exhausted me. He gave my arm a good brisk rubdown and checked pressure points to see if there was any reflex present yet.

Throughout the previous few days, my friends and contemporaries had me in their thoughts and prayers and kept a steady stream of emails and faxes coming to the hospital's patient care office. Printed messages were delivered to my room read to me; I have saved them in a memory box along with numerous get-well cards sent that first week. Personnel from the elementary schools where I taught had a "care tree" made up of folks who called Momma and Jaime to keep track of my condition, constantly wanting to know when they might be able to come visit.

It is interesting to me that as of today's date, I do not remember much of anything that occurred while I was first hospitalized. Of course, the limited amount my brain was able to process about what had occurred continued to cause me a great deal of stress and overwhelming despondency. I truly didn't understand what had happened to me other than the fact I was gravely ill and was not able to have any conversation with my family or the medical providers who were caring for me. I was terrified that things weren't ever going to be any different, that I would remain in that condition, and I kept asking God to just let me die.

Kay - my sister who lives the closest - was able to leave work and drive back to see me and check on my progress. She also helped keep everybody's spirits up, wouldn't let them get down in the dumps, and went with Momma to go pick up my baby boy at his daycare. My poor little guy was very confused. He had been told that Mama wasn't feeling good and would be home soon, but you can tell by looking at a picture taken of him at school 10 days after my stroke, he was one frightened and sad little boy.)

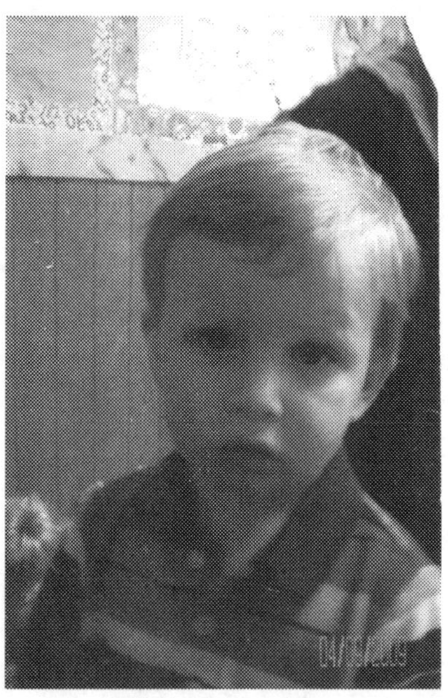

Little Blue Boy at Daycare, Age 2

By late afternoon on the fifth day of my hospitalization, I had not yet been seen by the associate of the doctor in charge of my case; Daddy decided to stand outside of my room and watch the nurses' station. About 5:00 p.m., he noticed a doctor he had not seen before talking to a staff member in the nurses working area. He surmised that this doctor was the one who was supposed to have been there earlier in the day to examine me. After about 20 minutes of watching and listening to what he determined was not a hospital-related conversation he approached the doctor, introduced himself as my father, and asked if he was there to examine me; he looked at his notes and replied that he was, but he couldn't do it because his laptop battery wasn't charged, and he had to return to his office for another one. Daddy told him that he would be there waiting for his return, and it didn't matter how long it took or how late it was, he intended to hear what a staff physician had to say about my present condition, and whether it had worsened or improved. Keep in mind, I had not had a **complete** physical evaluation by anybody since the "floating ER physician" was replaced five days earlier by hospital personnel.

The hospital associate doctor returned at 7:30 p.m. and Daddy and Jaime were there waiting for him. While they were outside my room Daddy told him how very disappointed the family was with the care that I had received thus far. He stated unequivocally that he intended for him to give me a comprehensive examination and write an evaluation before he left there that evening. Just to make sure there was no question, Daddy told him that every effort was being made to get me transferred, and that we needed a written record of his evaluation, detailing what had, or more importantly *had not been,* done for me during my stay at the hospital.

In about half an hour, the doctor came out and spoke with Daddy and Jaime about his findings during this examination. Daddy told him that his exam had been the first neurology unit staff's attention I had received since they took over my case and that he appreciated him doing it. The doctor was a little contrite saying he would have performed the same level of exam even if Daddy hadn't been so agitated.

The next day, when Jaime checked with our contact at Into The Light Stroke Rehabilitation Therapy Hospital (ITLRT), she told him that I could not be transferred there as long as I had any IV's or emergency medical equipment attached to my body. We informed the patient care office of this because the nurses on the floor I was on told Daddy they couldn't remove anything until a staff physician's final release was obtained. Further, the patient care office said I would have to be transferred out of my CCU into a room on a regular floor before **any** of this could happen. As 2:00 p.m. approached, we felt like the hospital was dragging its feet on my discharge and everybody was getting upset and annoyed again.

At 3 o'clock, two male nurses appeared at the door of my room and said they were there to move me; they got my paperwork together and wheeled me and my bed to a regular room and departed without another word. The final remaining thing that had to be taken care of was the removal of the cardio ventricular catheter in my right arm. In just a few minutes, a nurse we had never seen before showed up and said she was there to perform that task. Luckily, I did not watch, nor do I remember, that it was approximately 14 inches long and it was a very involved and painful procedure; it had stuck to my skin at the insertion point under my arm where it snaked through the vein to my heart. The nurse, who apparently didn't have experience removing this type of catheter, was nervous and shaky and apologized again and again because taking it out caused my arm to start bleeding and wasn't easily accomplished. Momma couldn't watch, but Jaime did, and he said it was really disturbing.

We had previously been told that the latest I would be accepted at Into The Light Hospital as a patient transfer was 5:00 p.m. and by now it was 4:15. We got in touch with our contact and she said the ITLRT ambulance transfer personnel were sitting outside my hospital at that very minute and that I would be accepted at their Emergency Room even if traffic on the way there slowed them down past the 5:00 p.m. deadline.

CHAPTER
Two

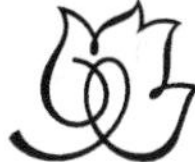

We collected my records and I was released from the hospital at 5:05 p.m. for a 45-minute ride to Into The Light Therapy Hospital. At last ...we were on our way to what we hoped would be dedicated attention to my condition.

Jaime followed the ambulance, Daddy and Kay went to pick up Brandon, and Momma went by the house to pick up items that I would need while a patient at Into The Light (ITLRT). By the time she found her way there it was after 7:00 p.m. and the outside doors were locked. Luckily, some people sitting in the lobby opened the doors from the inside, so she could get in and come see me in what was to be my “home away from home” for the next 61 days. I was sharing a corner room and bath with another patient, but my family didn’t care because I was finally where everybody thought I could get some help.

One of the things that nobody had taken into consideration during the frenetic struggle to get me out of one hospital and into another, was the fact that my mental condition was beyond broken. Everything was geared up to go, go, go and I could see no reason to live. After I was taken to my room, divided by a curtain for privacy, the check-in exams continued. A catheter was put in place without even asking my husband to leave the room, my bed adjusted to the technician's instructions, and all I could think of was that it was hopeless. I was lost again ...very sad. Since none of the doctors held a conversation with my parents in my presence, I still did not know what had happened to me and was terribly fearful and confused.

Early the next morning, alone except for a therapy technician, I again prayed to God to let me die ...I didn't want to go on ...in the prime of my life, every-thing was lost. About thirty minutes later, Dr. Bryan McCall looked in on me and introduced himself. He told me he would be heading up the team who would be working with me and that he would come back with each of the specialty therapists on Monday morning to get everything rolling. He told me to get some rest during the next two days because Monday we were "going to get to work." On Saturday and Sunday, I was given sponge baths in my bed and the appendages on my right side were massaged. On those two days, the head of my bed was elevated for me to eat my meals instead of swinging my legs off the bed.

As I was laying there with my eyes closed, Daddy, Momma and Kay came to visit; they were quietly talking about my condition because they thought I was asleep. All I could think was I wished I was dead. I could find no reason to live like that, not being able to speak, walk, remember ...anything! I spent most of my time sleeping because of the medications, which looking back, was great because that was the last day that would happen for as long as I was there. I kept my eyes shut and feigned being asleep, but all I could think about was how miserably unhappy I was. Fear of the unknown is a debilitating emotion that seriously ill people experience.

At 8 o'clock on Monday morning Jaime, his parents, Momma, Daddy, and Kay, all had the opportunity to be briefed on the direction the Rehabilitation Unit would be taking. Dr. McCall apologized because the weekend had interfered with us getting started on my rehab but assured everybody that we were going to "hit the ground running." Boy, was *that ever* the truth. Monday was a different story all the way around. An aide came in and helped me get into a special roll-around wheelchair used just in the bathroom; she gave me a shower and washed my hair and for the first time in almost a week I felt clean and "almost human" again. This was the first of many days that my personal care daily activity was conducted on a set schedule and according to accepted procedures.

Unfortunately, two of the aides who were assigned to take care of me were very curt and gave me the impression I was "putting them out," but one lady was extremely caring and sweet to me and I always hoped she would be on duty when it came time to move me to the bathroom.

I was really at the mercy of whoever showed up when I pushed the call button, because since I couldn't talk I was not able to tell them what I needed. The operator who sat at the desk would ask "Do you need any assistance" or "do you need somebody to come?" but I couldn't say anything in response. I was still limited to "I'm" or "My."

Something very scary happened about the fifth day there that involved one of the staff who did not follow the enforced safety procedure they used to help move patients around. A wide belt was strapped around my waist which gave them something substantial to lift with since I wasn't capable of standing up and moving around without falling. I had pushed the call button a couple of times because I needed assistance, and after several minutes, an unpleasant nurse's aide came in to help me. She was grumbling and rushing around; and when she grabbed the belt and pulled me up, she lost her balance and we both fell to the floor. She had already mumbled that I was too heavy to "deal with," so she blamed me after we fell.

That really frightened me, so I avoided going to go the bathroom for three days. There were "Use The Belt To Avoid Falls" posters everywhere, so I'm sure she got in trouble because it could have been very serious if I had broken a bone ...as it was, I had a large bruise on my hip for over a week. She never came back again after that when I pushed the call button for someone to help me.

The next aide that was assigned to my room was also brusque and not very caring, but I guess taking care of invalid people day in and day out hardens your heart and uses up all your patience.

Another assault on my sensibilities was the simple matter of brushing my teeth. I couldn't stand up in front of the sink to spit after brushing. The right side of my face was pulled down because of stroke paralysis, so I would dribble and slobber down the front of my gown. The occupational therapist who came in to help me get dressed each morning was always late picking me up, and when I would point to my gown she would just say, "Oh, it's okay" - when I knew it certainly was not and was terribly embarrassed because I knew I needed washing off.

We settled into a routine very quickly – I was allowed to eat my meals sitting up in bed, and was encouraged to rest; but speech, occupational and physical therapists came to my room throughout the day and got me up and into my chair for the various exercises. On Wednesday mornings throughout my stay there, staff met with family members to let everybody know the progress that was being made. I'll have to admit that after my therapy sessions started, I had little time to dwell on my broken life, and whatever antidepressants they were giving me took the edge off my sorrow.

Every morning a nurse came in and performed a blood stick to make sure my blood count wasn't heading toward diabetes since the prednisone they were giving me to help speed the healing process could possibly cause me to become diabetic. Every day she would ask me my name in an attempt for me to talk to her. We were overjoyed about 10 days later when I could tell her my name was Kiir.

After 14 days, Dr. McCall ordered an articulated leg/ foot brace be made to fit me. It arrived in about a week and I began the job of learning to walk with assistance. Soon after, it was decided that I was strong enough to be wheeled down to the therapy floor where various physical therapists helped me stand up and take steps while I held on to a ballet bar, sit on thick foam mats and exercise my arm, go to speech therapy, and go into social interaction therapy groups.

It has been proven that singing is successful therapy to help stroke patients talk, and card/game playing helps the brain process numbers and reasoning skills in an informal atmosphere. Daddy and Momma would come in and we would play UNO with the therapist and another patient, so that was enjoyable. However, one of the saddest things that stands out in my memory is one day during our singing group session when Daddy and Momma were invited to sit in and sing along. The second song that we sang was "You Are My Sunshine," which is one that both my parents used to sing to me when I was little, and, as a matter of fact even after I was eight or nine years old. In the middle of the song, I looked up and there were tears in Daddy's eyes and Momma had to get up and leave because she was visibly crying. I hadn't been singing along up to that point, but I remember that day I sang the whole song.

For the most part, it was hard for me to come to grips with what the occupational therapists were trying to do for me, using shapes tests and puzzles exercises, because many were identical to those I used in my special education diagnostic testing. Luckily, I was fortunate to have very caring and knowledgeable people working to help me progress. I had my favorites who were especially kind to me.

Probably the most exhausting exercise I had to do was walking on a treadmill while hooked up to a parachute harness apparatus hung from a brace on the ceiling. It was a big leather belt that was secured around my midsection, with attached straps between my legs; it was hoisted up tight by a pully until my feet bore minimum weight. When the treadmill was turned on, the person on my left side moved my left leg forward, and alternatively, another therapist on my right side moved that leg forward which simulated me “walking”. The first day the time was for 3 minutes and we did it twice a day.

The second day it was 4 minutes each time. Each day after that they increased the minutes until we were up to 10 minutes. This was very difficult and uncomfortable but helped my brain re-learn that there were two legs that needed to take steps to walk. It seemed like it had been weeks since this trial began, but it was only but 8 days before I could move along on the treadmill at a quick pace for 15 minutes. Amazing!

As soon as that mountain was climbed, I was taken back over to the parallel bars that were 10 feet long and told to walk (of course, a therapist was right in front of me on a rolling stool). After three weeks of trying to master taking steps again, I was absolutely overjoyed the day I could walk the distance of those bars, go around the end of them and make the trip back to the starting point. Several of the daily therapy assistants were watching and gave me a round of applause. I remember thinking to myself – *You Did It, You Did It!*

Each day as I was secured in my wheelchair and moved from my room to the therapy floor, I was concentrating on what I might do to push the boundaries to get out of it! I couldn't imagine being in that situation any longer than necessary. Fortunately, because of good core strength, balance, and a strong left leg – all a direct result of 20 years of dance – plus a positive "never-give-up, keep-on-trying" mindset - I was able to discontinue using the chair much sooner than most ...but I'm getting ahead of myself, that's later, further down the road.

From then on, my daily progress was recorded by the number of steps I could take in a lap around the gym, or changing the cadence by making a round trip down the hall. Sometimes a therapy tech would accompany me or sometimes Momma, Daddy or Jaime. It was hard work, but I knew I was building muscles and stamina, so I made sure I gave it my best effort.

The same was true for my Occupational Therapy where they worked on getting my right arm loosened up, but at the same time it necessitated me using my left arm and hand which were not dominant. In the mornings, the OT would come in and make me learn how to put on my bra with one hand; she would also watch me put on my socks and shoes; comb and brush my hair; put on lipstick and mascara; pull up shorts or jeans and then pull up zippers or button buttons. So many daily activities that we take for granted once we are out of our toddler years are very nearly impossible to do if you only have the use of one hand, arm, and leg. Imagine how embarrassed I was after I had tried and failed to accomplish a task and buzzed for one of the aides to come help. When she got there, I pantomimed what I needed her to assist me with (since I wasn't able to talk at all); she looked at me with incredulity and said, "don't you remember how to use this?" and then, "can't you do anything?" Unfortunately, I didn't, and couldn't - not while balancing on one leg and using one hand, both on the left side of my body. I've talked to many people after

4 or 5 years that couldn't understand how I could have done many of these routine activities. In thinking about it, I finally figured out why I didn't have more problems than I did; I was born ambidextrous and routinely used to switch hands while writing, playing tennis, bowling, hammering in a nail, playing pool, etc., so as I relearned all my tasks again, it was almost natural to use my left hand. This is one more God given talent that has helped me in my recovery effort.

On the positive side, my OT used a EASU Stimulation (Electric Arm Stimulating Unit) device to help me open my hand 10 or 12 times a session. It gave me a big smile to see my hand move rather than be balled into a fist. This exercise enabled me to pick up rubber blocks and move them from one place to another. My therapist stressed that I had to strive every day to achieve small victories towards recovery. That made me realize that taking "baby steps" every day equaled mastering a therapy at the end of a week.

One of my favorite exercises was when I would sit down on a motorized bench and they would secure me onto it with a seatbelt; then the bench would slowly move up and forward until I was in a standing position with a tray in front of me. I usually stood in an upright position for 15 minutes, but sometimes longer if I felt like it. This was to keep my circulatory system working efficiently and to insure I had blood flow in my right leg and foot. It felt good to be upright even if I wasn't going anywhere.

Another exercise I had to do almost every day was to sit on a recumbent bike with my feet strapped to the pedals and they timed me while I pedaled like mad. If I didn't use both legs the monitor would alert to that, so the therapists would make me slow down and concentrate on using my right leg as well as my left. Those therapists were tough, but caring, and helped me immeasurably with my progress; they often joked around with me and said I was just a slacker and they were going to increase my torture to two hours instead of one. Even though I still could not have a real conversation with them, they knew what I was saying. One of the funny guys who was nicknamed "Pork-Chop" told me he didn't care how many dirty looks I gave him, he was going to make sure I could run a marathon before I left that hospital

Each day all of my assigned therapists and their assistants wrote a report or filled out a chart that was added to a notebook of my daily activities. That way, an analysis could be made at the end of the week to see what accomplishments I had made or what areas needed to be concentrated on the next week. Every two weeks Dr. McCall would call in patients for an informal interview and go over the progress charts. An excellent casual tool for him to see firsthand how patients were doing. During one of these chats he determined something he thought was relevant and that he was actively trying to resolve. Shortly thereafter he had his nurse come to my room to tell Daddy and Momma he'd like to see them in his office. When they got there, he asked if they were pleased with the therapy I was receiving, liked the hospital, and so forth. He then told them what he had discovered about my behavior; he reported that when he asked me if I am doing well, I always nod my head, reply in the affirmative, and am upbeat; when he asked me if my therapy is successful, I nod and smile; when he quickly changed the subject, and asked how many fingers he was holding up (e.g., either 2 or 3) I might say 4, or maybe 1. He then figured out that I was especially good at not being forthcoming or honest. He told them he had changed tactics with me because he wondered if my cognition might not be as good as he thought or perhaps I really didn't understand the question. Another suspicion, and the one he believed to be right, might be that out of self-preservation I was being extremely tricky and utilizing a defense mechanism that some stroke patients use to cover up their weakness. He went on to say this is a deep-seated ploy even demonstrated by animals who are injured. He ended by saying he wanted to let them know that it was possible I wasn't quite as far along as we thought and to be on the lookout. At Last!! I truly was in a facility where doctors were actively thinking and working towards a measurable recovery.

Through all my therapy sessions, I still was not able to converse other than saying a limited number of words. Extremely frustrating for everybody concerned but especially for me, a person whose life had changed so drastically and who had no way of knowing if I would ever approach living a normal life again. My Daddy bought a laptop to assist me in relaying my concerns, but I was not mentally able to use it. Jaime decided that I could use my son's magnetic ABC and numbers board which had a reverse white board with markers to remember/practice with. At that point in time I could not use it either because I still couldn't speak. Most of the time I was encouraged and felt my quality of life was improving, yet I still experienced deep black periods of not caring if I lived or died. ***However, through all of this, Jaime was there every day, day in and day***

out, from 8:00 in the morning until 10:00 at night. If there was ever a Rock of Gibraltar, he was it.

I do know, without a doubt, if it hadn't been for him, I would not have had the desire or strength to go on. I loved him and loved my little boy beyond measure, but I had no way of knowing if I would be able to be a *real* mother, a loving wife, or have a fulfilling life ever again. In just an instant, all of my hopes and dreams had disappeared like a puff of smoke.

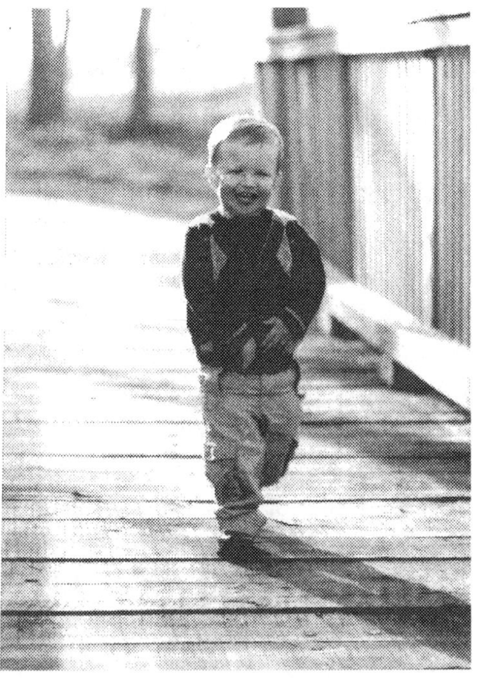

Brandon, age 2, walking in park

CHAPTER Three

After I had been in the Into The Light Therapy Rehab facility about three weeks, a private room became available and I moved into it – this made me very happy because I now had a little privacy and had my own bathroom! As sometimes happens, along with good things, you must accept the bad. On that wing of the floor, one of the aides was dismissive and insulting about having to clean me up. I really wanted to tell her I'd rather have anything in the world happen other than for her to do that ...but it was still physically impossible for me to speak at that point, so I couldn't tell her so. An adult woman who must rely on somebody to wash her like a baby learns how much she has taken for granted. I had never been so demoralized in my life. I'd always been a very modest person and every bit of privacy and dignity were stripped away daily. It would be cathartic now to have the opportunity to tell that aide how damaging she was, and what a negative effect it had on an already-fragile psyche.

There were three other aides on that area of the floor who seemed to enjoy taking advantage of someone they had control of by insulting or demeaning them. This never happened when Jamie was within earshot or when Momma was in the room; since they knew communication was an issue, there was no way for them to be held accountable and they knew it. If Momma smiled and was friendly to one of my tormentors, I'd scowl or wave my hand in a negative manner; when the aide left, Momma would urge me to be "nice" instead of acting "ugly". It was only after I could fully explain my feelings a year later that my mother understood what I had been trying to relay to her. If the hospital and family members only knew what a negative effect those personnel have on the patients, they would see that they were relegated to making beds or mopping floors.

I had been asking Jamie to bring Brandon to see me so I could hold my little boy, and pretty soon Dr. McCall gave us permission for him to come up on a weekend when tasks not directly involving patient care were going on. So, on a Sunday, about five weeks after my stroke, Jamie, Brandon, and Momma came for a visit. Since the 29th of March, when Brandon had asked his Daddy where Mama was, he had been telling him that I was very sick; as they were walking down the hall to my room I could see him peering in each door that was open and when they entered mine and he saw me sitting in my tall hospital bed, he was a little afraid. He came to me very slowly at first but then was happy to see his Mama and wanted to crawl all over me and the bed. I cried with happiness to be able to have my precious boy on my lap again.

Jamie brought him again the next week, and this time I was sitting in my wheelchair. He thought it was great fun to push me down the hall, through the therapy room and out the door onto the terrace for our visit. The fish in the aquarium in the gym also kept him entertained when he wasn't "driving" me around. Amazingly, I remembered my own interaction with fish at the private school so many years before; I couldn't remember much else, but seeing him walking back and forth talking to the fish sparked that memory in my subconscious. Momma saw my eyes sparkling and patting my chest saying "me" and patting the side of the tank and knew what I was thinking.

It wasn't too long after that when I started my water therapy in the deep pool. It involved a therapist helping me get out of my wheelchair into a pneumatic chair lift that swung out over the pool, then lowered me and the chair all the way down into the water. At the time, Jamie, Mom, Dad and Kay all thought that I was really enjoying the water exercises because I would open my mouth and say "Oh, Oh, Oh, and they said my eyes were big and excited. It wasn't until months later that I told them I was absolutely petrified. I had no idea if I could walk with a cane up and down the pool or whether my leg would just collapse and I'd go underwater! It did give me an opportunity to walk weightless and let my right leg and foot become accustomed to the sensation of moving along in a normal gait. Even though I understood, finally, it was good for me, I never got past the idea that I couldn't swim and that I might drown. My mind had not yet caught up with some of the things my body could do already. The minute I was discharged, the water therapy ended, and I was a little saddened then. Momma offered to suit up and get in with me, but we never had the opportunity since Day Neuro didn't have that included as part of my regimen. But here I am getting a little ahead of myself again.

All therapies continued every day: I began at 7:00 and continued until 11:30 when I came back to my room for lunch and a nap, then began again at 1:30 and ended at 4:00. Much emphasis was put on the necessity that I sleep so my brain could rest. Unfortunately, that was when my friends from work wanted to come see me. I had visitors very regularly, so many that I started telling Jamie and Momma that I didn't want to see anybody. Folks still came, which let me know that everybody was concerned about me. Teachers from one of the schools where I previously taught classes had a prayer blanket made for me that had pictures and prayers sewn on it. Friends and associates from three other schools in the district took turns coming on a bi-weekly basis. There was always a friendly face or two there, encouraging me to get better quickly. In addition, a group of them got together and collected money to purchase a play station for me; part of the package included both physical and mental games for me to play after I was released from the hospital. What a wonderful bunch of friends. I hope I made it clear enough that they understood how grateful I was for their thoughtfulness and generosity. There never was a time that I didn't have at least two flower arrangements to brighten my room and lots and lots of get-well cards taped to the wall. Jamie brought pictures of Brandon, and my sweet "Other Mother" brought a picture board of snapshots of Jamie and me, so I had constant reminders of my loving little family.

During those weeks, Ann, Kay and Aunt Victoria took turns coming in on week-end visits to see me, and that gave Brandon some interface with family other than Momma. She would leave every day about 3:00 o'clock to avoid the traffic on the freeway and would pick him up and take him home. When my sisters and auntie were here, they would try to go someplace fun with my little guy, or just stay home and play with him. Everybody was very concerned about the effect my not being at home was having on him. His forward-thinking and attentive pediatrician told Momma that even though it might not manifest itself for a year, or much later, this would eventually have a traumatic effect on him, i.e., separation anxiety.

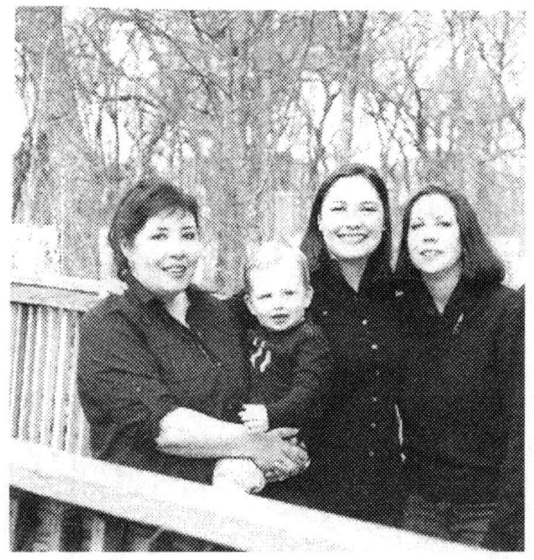

Auntie Ann, Cousin Leigh, Auntie Kay

Momma spent as much time as she could with me, and she and Brandon were together a great deal of the time, becoming very close. Even though she tried every night to get him to go to sleep in his bed – or in her bed – he waited until Jamie got home to go to sleep. It was kind of like "you and me against the world, Daddy."

When Momma went back home to be with Daddy every three or four weeks, my two Godsends -Anna (Other Mother) and DeWitt (Dad^2)-stepped in and took care of little Brandon, insuring that he got to and from day-school every day, and making life as normal as possible at Grandma and Granddad's house. Anna told me that even though Brandon would be sleepy after his dinner and bath, he insisted on waiting for Jamie to get home from the hospital before he would get in the "big bed" to go to sleep. This was the start of him staying up late every night instead of going to sleep at 7:00 o'clock like he used to do with me. To this day, he doesn't want to go to sleep until 11:00 p.m.

Another important part of my life that took a while for me to remember was my pet kitty-cat. He was a beautiful white Turkish Angora that I bought as a kitten in 1997, and his name was Snowman. Young women are usually crazy about their cats and I certainly was no exception ...we loved each other. He spent every minute with me when I was home, was amazingly vocal, and was very smart. He could sense when I was sad, happy, or just wanted to "chill out"; whatever the mood, he was there. He slept in my lap when I watched TV, on the carpet in the bathroom when I bathed to get ready to leave, on the foot of my bed on a faux fur throw at night, and if I left town to visit my parents he went along with me in the car. A positively adored pet. The morning of my stroke he was agitated and meowing as if he was afraid for me. Jaime said he would run in the living room when he got home from the hospital to see if I had come back with him. So, there was no surprise that he had missed me terribly and never left my side after I returned home following my long hospital stay. We resumed our close friendship with him filling his role as constant companion; I don't doubt that his "offering his back" for me to rub probably helped with my emotional recovery. No questions asked, just unfaltering love. The 2nd of May was his 19th birthday and he had all the ailments that old cats come down with: he was almost blind in both eyes, he was deaf for all practical purposes, his teeth were loose and 2 of them had fallen out, and the little cysts that he had developed on his belly were diagnosed as fast-growing cancers. So, in May of 2016, I was forced into the hardest decision I ever made when I had to have him put to sleep. He had been there for me, but I had to let him go, and it was a painful goodbye.

CHAPTER
Four

I kept making daily progress with my rehabilitation and got to the point that the occupational therapist thought I could leave the hospital and go to an off-site salon where I could get my nails done and have a pedicure. Oh, what an adventure that was for me, and something that let me know I was making gains towards getting back into the real world. It was so good to get outside again.

I had a couple of heart monitoring tests that lasted a week each time, and had an extensive eye exam to ascertain if any lasting damage had been done by the stroke. Much to my relief, I passed both these tests with flying colors.

As the days went by and I could perform my therapies easier, the nurses and therapists kept mentioning that it wouldn't be long before I would be discharged. Jamie told them he wanted to bring me home some weekend for a furlough, so I could reacquaint myself with my old surroundings, figure out how I could manage going to the bathroom, how to get up on our tall bed, or simply propel myself around the corners of the house in my wheelchair. He admitted to our nurse that he was apprehensive about how he could handle me at home without her on stand-by. My husband had been such a stalwart caregiver that I never knew he had misgivings. He wasn't the only one - I was very concerned about what would happen when we were home alone.

The big day came, and with a nurse helping Jamie get me into the car and buckled in, we both allowed ourselves to smile. The trip up the toll road was frightening with all the traffic racing by, and when we got on the turnpike I had no recollection of where we were going. As we exited the IH and turned onto the connector loop Jamie asked me if I knew where we were. I just shook my head no. Overwhelming to realize all my short-term memory was completely gone! I did not recognize our street when we turned on it, did not recognize the house when we drove up, nor did I remember the interior of the house when he wheeled me inside. I thought to myself that it was pretty and had nice colors, but I did not know that I had decorated and re-painted everything myself just a week before my stroke.

Anna was there with Brandon, waiting for us to get settled, and she recognized that I was confused and was having trouble remembering. Brandon was acting afraid and didn't want to be around me. This was not, in any way, a successful homecoming. Looking back now, I remember these things happening, and how disturbed I was because I was in a place that I had absolutely no connection to – all associated memories were lost until my brain had time to heal. I enjoyed the time being away from the ITLRT hospital and with the family, so it was bittersweet when I had to return to the facility on Sunday night.

I had three such furloughs and was more at ease each time, twice spending an afternoon on my chair and ottoman. My Other Mother made sure there was food to eat and snacks to enjoy. I was becoming very concerned about what would happen when I came home for good and had to manage trips to the bathroom, showers, shampooing my hair, and all regular daily activities, without oversight. It seemed to all of us that I still needed the safety of being a patient in the hospital to get better, but I had made such rapid progress the insurance company didn't see it that way. We were informed that my discharge was scheduled to take place on June 6th.

As the date approached, I became even more disturbed about whether or not I could truly take care of myself at home. The thought of navigating my wheelchair around the corners, narrow halls, doorways and bathrooms in the house was making me very anxious. I was dependent on a member of the hospital care staff being with me to monitor my medicine and help avoid accidents in the bathroom. More angst over things I was no longer comfortable with.

One day, Momma and Daddy questioned a nurse in the neurological care office about the possibility of me transferring to a therapy/limited nursing care facility before I made the giant step to be on my own at home. She gave them the names of two residential therapy centers that were designed for either short or long-term care. The first was a foster home arrangement; the physical therapy program was set up to assist the elderly versus active exercising, so that one was off the list even though it was attractive, clean, and smelled good. The second was 40 miles from the house, but during the long drive out Momma was trying to remain optimistic. The information brochure had nice pictures of private rooms, it mentioned arts and crafts facilities, covered pavilions for picnics, walking paths that accommodated wheelchairs, communal dining rooms, card playing areas, and more importantly, a well-equipped therapy/gym area with the latest equipment and hot tubs; everything geared to assist patients' recovery as quickly as possible. All-in-all, it sounded too good to be true. When they arrived, and pulled into a large parking area, there were various choices and they decided to park next to one of the residential cottages. The entrance door opened directly into the living room; when they went inside there were several residents who had varying degrees of disabilities watching television. One of them asked Momma if she had come to see her. Another one asked if it was time for lunch (this was 3 o'clock in the afternoon). A cursory walk-through the cottage showed several residents in bed, staring at the ceiling. Very depressing. A quick stop by the Welcome Center was more like the brochure pictures, but the "happy place" facility and camaraderie they hoped to find was nowhere to be seen. The trip home was silent for the most part. After getting over the disappointment of not finding a good halfway house for me to transition to, they decided that my own comfortable home was the best place for me, and where my mental recovery could best begin. So, June 13, 2009, I came home to start working on my new life.

CHAPTER *Five*

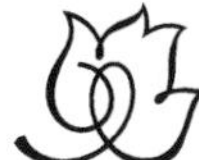

Before I left the ITLRT facility, I had a one-on-one meeting with Dr. McCall. He was basically being a *cheerleader*, encouraging me to look at the upcoming change as a whole new life, a chance to excel, and an opportunity to relearn as many things as I could when I was back in the comfort of my own home. Of course, he warned me about things that might be dangerous, but he stressed that I push the envelope to see what I could do. He said the word ***can't*** should not be part of my vocabulary. He also said, **"don't cry Uncle"** until you have proven to yourself that whatever you are trying to do should only be put on a back burner until you're a little stronger and surer of your surroundings.

One of the things he highly recommended was for me to encourage Jaime to be intimate again. He pointed out that we were both in our thirties and in the prime of our lives. Prior to my stroke, I enjoyed making love and it was a very important part of our marriage. Now, I wasn't open to this suggestion because I felt like I was no longer desirable. I didn't have romantic feelings because I was very self-conscious about the paralysis in my arm and the inability to use my right leg. I couldn't fathom my husband wanting to make love with me. This was another thing on my long list of heart-breaking disappointments that I didn't think would ever be overcome. Dr. McCall sent me off with a hug and the advice to not give up on Jamie and me. (Point of Interest: One entire year passed before I was emotionally able to enjoy our physical relationship again, causing an underlying strain in our relationship.)

About a month after my stroke, Momma hired a recommended cleaning service to come by the house once a week to keep up with basic housework. She didn't have time to do that plus make daily visits to the hospital and take care of Brandon. They did an adequate job, so she called them again to come give the house a thorough going-over before my discharge and homecoming. When I came home, it was to a clean, nice-smelling house, and Momma had washed everything, and my clothes were folded and put away.

For all our trepidation, moving back home was nerve-racking but it basically went off without a hitch. I was *very* excited! About the only thing that was an issue was getting to the bathroom during the night. First, I had to get out of bed without falling on my nose, get into my wheelchair with Jaime's help, put on my sock, brace and tennis shoe, and then finally he would push me into the bathroom and position the wheeler close to the "potty room" door. I then had to stand, pivot out of the wheelchair and onto the commode without anything to hold onto. The procedure to get up and back into my wheelchair was even more difficult because of restricted maneuvering room and me having to just use my left arm and leg to accomplish the task. It goes without saying that this function took some time, so it couldn't be decided on at the last minute. Just another thing that I had always taken for granted. And it was a task that puts strain on the lives of the people involved: love, honor, and obey doesn't normally include physically handling your partner for middle of the night potty runs.

That being said, I thanked God every night for giving me the strength to be able do this necessary task. I can only imagine how difficult it would be for an elderly couple to accomplish the same thing; I don't believe it could be done, so what is the answer for them?

I came home on a Thursday, and the following Monday I showed up at the Day Neuro Outpatient Center, starting the newest part of my therapy to help me cope with everyday life. Even though they had the group doing some basic exercises, my first activity was drying and folding towels, a little walking on a treadmill, simple word exercises and common-sense problem solving; I didn't think it was really the kind of help that I needed but they have that protocol set up for everybody so that was where I started. The speech problem was still insurmountable because I couldn't voice my desires, thoughts, and fears – truthfully, unable to communicate much of anything. The procedure that was in place was for me to point at workbook pictures and they would guess what I wanted to say. Many times, I could repeat the word they said, but just as often I could not.

I did enjoy crafts therapy - it was very relaxing to me and I was able to focus on being creative and painting instead of having to worry about talking. A colorful painted glass sun catcher of a tiger that I made in crafts therapy is now a permanent decoration in our kitchen window, still catching the sun's rays and reminding me of "when".

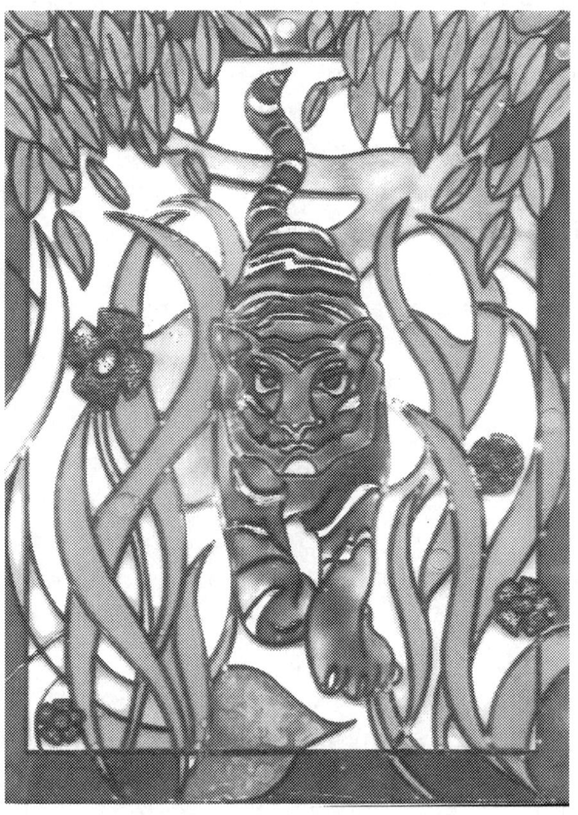

Tiger Sun Catcher

While I was there, the therapists accompanied me to the Center's cafeteria where I picked out my own lunch and paid for it. Another time, they took me to a mall for a little shopping. Momma made sure I had some money in my purse so I could buy something ...of course, that first purchase was a lime green shirt with a whale on it for my precious little boy.

The Day Neuro therapy was not authorized by my insurance company for very long; the next step for me was to get scheduled as quickly as possible to take part in a Home Therapy Program. Occupational/Speech/ physical therapists were to come to my house for sessions versus being in a hospital environment; this was set up to help disassociate real life from patient care.

CHAPTER
Six

Three days before the in-home therapy was scheduled to commence, the unthinkable happened. I had been feeling very tired and lethargic every day after coming home from therapy, basically sleeping the afternoons away. Jaime mentioned this to one of the Day Neuro staff administrators who checked with the doctor. My charts were carefully reviewed and three of the side effects of the anti-seizure medication I was taking are sleepiness, lethargy, and dizziness. It was an R_X originally prescribed by an ER doctor from the other hospital 12 weeks earlier, so it was decided that I should quit taking it on a trial basis to see if that alleviated the problem of my being so tired.

After two days of feeling a little dizzy and headachy - and telling the staff at Day Neuro a couple of times so they would make a record of it for the trial period - on Friday, July 1ST, I suffered a grand mal seizure. When we got home that afternoon, I told Jaime I wasn't feeling very well and that I wanted to take a shower and wash my hair before going to bed. He got me situated in the shower and was sitting on the bed about 12 feet away, watching TV while waiting for me to finish. In just a few minutes he heard a loud crash and ran in the bathroom where he found me face down in the shower. I was unconscious, my paralyzed leg tucked beneath me, and the chair turned over between me and the back wall.

He yelled at Momma to come, but she was giving Brandon a bath and had to get him out of the tub. In the minute or so that it took her to get to my bathroom, I had started turning blue. Jaime told her to call 911, they answered immediately, and the operator told Momma to get me in a sitting position. Since I was down, wet, and soapy in the shower, this just wasn't possible. Jaime and Momma both tried and tried to get me up or on my side where I could breathe, but weren't totally successful; the best that they could do was get me on my side. The 911 Operator was waiting on the phone the whole time and told Momma that the ambulance was outside the house. Luckily, it was the same crew that had responded when I had my stroke, so they knew their way in and had me up and out of the shower very quickly. By that time, I had regained consciousness. Poor Brandon had been abandoned in the living room and he was standing there with a towel hanging around his head. He hadn't moved from where Momma left him, so he was right in the middle of the chaotic scene until she got back to carry him away from the area. Traumatic for a 2-year old, to say the least.

It had probably been 10 minutes before EMS arrived and another 15 before they wheeled me out to the ambulance. The crew was trying to keep me upbeat and not so frightened so one of them jokingly said "ready to roll Lady Godiva?" because all I had on was my little diamond stud earrings. Once again, I was alone in an ambulance, totally terrified, wondering if this was another stroke and if I was going to die, *why, why, why?*

Jamie called his mother and asked her to please come and take care of Brandon; unfortunately, it was right in the middle of rush hour on the turnpike, so she couldn't get across town to the house until about six o'clock. She had called DeWitt, who arrived at the hospital shortly after I did, but since I was in the critical care emergency room they wouldn't let him in.

Momma and Jaime were both absolutely scared to death because they thought I'd had another stroke. Before leaving the house, he started for the car two or three times, but his legs were shaking so bad he couldn't walk and had to kneel on the floor. Momma just held Brandon close to her and they watched *Dora The Explorer* to keep him busy.

After Jamie calmed down just a little bit and left for the hospital, Momma called Daddy, Ann, and Kay to let them what had happened and promised she would call back and give them an update as soon as she had something to report. My Other Mother got to the house in record time considering all roads were jammed with 5 o'clock traffic. Momma was getting a delayed start, so she was waiting to leave the minute Anna arrived; it had been an hour since Jaime left so by the time she got to the hospital, it had already been determined that I had not suffered another stroke, but rather it was a grand mal seizure. Nothing to be discounted but not as life threatening as a stroke so that was good news.

Momma was upset that the ambulance took me back to the same hospital where we had to fight to get me discharged, but apparently EMS is required to transport patients to the nearest hospital when they are in critical condition. At any rate, I was admitted once again to a stroke floor room where they started running tests to try to ascertain what had happened. Momma called Dr. Tim Moe's office and learned he was out of town for the 4TH of July weekend, but the answering service said they would inform his associate who would check on me. That doctor (Dr. Myles Miller) returned her call the next day and said he would go by the hospital that afternoon to look over the test results.

The ER had done an MRI which indicated with certainty that I had not had a stroke, and on Saturday morning they ran an EEG to check brainwave activity. The young staff neurologist told Momma that some differences in recent brain activity indicated a seizure, but nothing was presenting at the time the EEG was made, so it was hard to know why it occurred. When we asked what might have contributed to the cause, he told us that 18% of stroke patients also have seizures at some later date. This same doctor also mentioned that the MRI indicated some peripheral blood flow had been restored on the left side of my brain. We have never found out what this might indicate, if anything.

Point of Interest: We are all wondering why nobody thought it might be a good thing for families of stroke victims to know to be alert to the fact that seizures might occur.

When Dr. Miller arrived a short time later, checked my chart and saw my status, he suggested that since it was the 4TH of July weekend with only a skeleton staff working, and no other tests were going to be run, he thought we might want to go home. He made an appointment for me to come see him at his office the following Thursday and left orders for the hospital to release me and send some anti-seizure medication home with me. Once again, we had a big scare ...*What on earth was going on?*

CHAPTER Seven

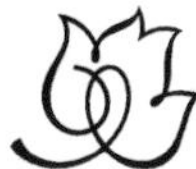

After ten days and a follow-up exam in Dr. Miller's office, he released me to return to Day Neuro and the program previously set up for me started again. However, only two weeks later (incredible, since it was almost immediately after a troubling set-back like suffering the seizure, and 10 days of recovery therapy) my insurance company said it was time to stop the Day Neuro level of rehab. It's not very heart-warming to realize that an insurance administrator sitting hundreds of miles away can dictate treatment for someone who is trying with all their might to recover from life-altering events. Jaime called and had several conversations with those people, but it was to no avail - the computer had made the decision. We were concerned about this "brush off" by the insurance company, and we were apprehensive about the credentials of someone coming to the house to perform my speech, physical and occupational therapies. It seemed to all of us that I still needed the safety of being in a hospital environment to get better.

As it turned out, our fears were totally unfounded: I was introduced to two of the most knowledgeable and caring therapists that I had encountered to that point. The first was my speech therapist Georgia, and the second was physical therapist Carin. I made more progress with Georgia in six weeks than I did the whole time I was a patient at the stroke therapy facility. We all, of course, had been told that my problems with speech were aphasia, apraxia and dysarthria. However, knowing those limitations and totally understanding the physical problem had never been thoroughly explained. Georgia provided us with that information which was both good and bad news because of the severity of dealing with all three. After our first session at home with her, she instructed Momma to buy a pad of adhesive labels and print the name of everything in the house I encountered. Washing machine, dryer, door, cabinet, refrigerator, stove, coffee pot, mirror, sofa, bed, dresser, toilet paper, telephone, picture of Jaime, everything I touched should have its name stuck to it. Her therapy motto was, "see it, say it, spell it, you own it!" This started me down the right track and gave me a tool that got me started talking again!

Carin and I established a wonderful rapport and she had me doing things that no one had even approached before. She worked on my gait, posture and core strength. Each visit I was becoming more and more sure of my ability to walk without fear, and my self-confidence returned very quickly, whereas before I had been tentative and afraid that I was going to fall.

Several months passed and when Daddy and Momma came for their monthly visit, I told them I wanted to try to drive again. I had been very critical of everybody's driving and one-day Momma had remarked that she would be very happy for me to drive again so she could complain to me about how badly I drove ...I replied, "Me too!" I had already approached her about this possibility during a phone conversation she and I had before they drove in. I just felt like I had recovered enough mobility that I wanted to at least try, and I wanted them to think about it and discuss it on the way to my house.

Since my parents have always encouraged me to try anything I think I can do, they agreed to drive my car over to a big (unopened) Big Box parking lot to see if my driving was even a possibility. Momma got in the passenger seat with her hand on the parking brake, and Daddy got in the back and leaned through the seats while I settled in the driver's seat for the first time in more than 8 months. I put my left foot on the accelerator and inched forward about 6 feet ...then stopped and inched forward 20 feet ...then stopped and backed up 10 feet. Then stopped, started off slowly and drove the length of one row before stopping again. They were laughing, I was laughing. Then I just put my head down on the steering wheel and cried. Oh, what an exhilarating feeling! Free again.

With a little more practice, my confidence grew, and I was ready to go home; I drove right up to the house and smoothly into our driveway. After taking a short break for refreshments, it was time to go again. I said, "Okay – we need to go to FedMart!" and off we went. I was too nervous to even think about getting on the freeway, so we drove only on back roads to get there. That was truly a "red letter day" on my journey back to being *me*. From then on, going to Chanteclaire, Northwest Center, Albany, the grocery store, the service station for gas, *wherever*, **I** drove! As I said earlier, just learn to believe ...God works in strange and wonderful ways.

Daddy had done a lot of computer research on a new Electronic Stimulation (E-STEM) system called Bionic, and we requested one from ITLST facility be brought to the house. Although it wasn't a system Carrin was completely familiar with, she began my therapeutic use of the Bionic unit. The day she put it on me and the unit helped me walk back and forth the length of my living room, I screamed with joy! This was another milestone day.

But, the Bionic proved to be both a blessing and a curse because it removed me from the umbrella of ITLST care as they did not actively use or promote the Bionic. My insurance company approved the use of the unit, but that meant I had to transfer to a regional hospital about 22 miles away to receive training on how to use the device and to receive actual therapy with the unit. This transfer meant leaving Georgia as well. More changes ...seemed at the time like it might not be worth it, but God continually offers us more rivers to cross. Another big adjustment to make at the start of 2010.

CHAPTER *Eight*

2010 Changing to the new hospital did not go without a hitch. Being able to make appointments with occupational, physical and speech therapists on the same day approached being a "too-hard-to-do" task. After 2 weeks, we finally got started on a routine that necessitated a 44-mile round trip 3 times a week. The ELSU therapy is one that they routinely use at that hospital, and the two physical therapists I saw regularly were very good. The two occupational therapists were very knowledgeable and worked diligently to help me recover use of my arm (the OT who had worked with me previously hadn't helped much at all; she just helped me fold towels and put sheets on the bed – which is important but there is much more to daily living than that). The new aggressive therapy at the different hospital was a pleasant surprise and gave me some hope that my arm might be of use again. They used a lot of vibration stimuli up and down the back of my hand and arm that pinpointed where feeling was returning. Daddy ordered a mirror box therapy device from England; I would look in a mirror at the back of the closed box to watch my good hand moving, and my fisted right hand would try to make the same movement. Both exciting and interesting to learn that the left side of my brain was trying to take over the activities that the right side could no longer perform. Also, there were numerous ball grasping and moving exercises that my brain had to really concentrate on and work hard at to make it happen. Progress again measured in baby steps.

I had pool therapy with a great OT who would get in the water with me and help with stretching and reaching exercises which pleased us all. Then, an unannounced personnel change occurred and everything kind of fell apart. The OT who started overseeing my pool therapy was afraid of the water (that certainly didn't seem logical) so she never got in with me. She only sat on the edge and timed exercises shown in a book, or had me walk on a submerged treadmill for five or six minutes. These changes were very disappointing for both me and my parents.

Additionally, after being there 6 weeks we were notified that my insurance company wouldn't continue to pay for my ELSU leg therapy past 45 days since they deemed it experimental. The Bionic unit was very expensive, so before we purchased one my therapist told Momma that we could "try out" a unit for 30 days. Since I seemed to be making good progress, of course my mother talked to the Bionic Corporate representative and ordered one for me.

Unfortunately, we also were **not** told ahead of time that once the unit arrived and was set up to my specifications, after 2 weeks the hospital physical therapist would no longer be authorized to lead me through my regular weekly therapy sessions. A real Catch-22. On the plus side, I was given a sense of freedom since I no longer had to wear an articulated brace and use a cane. My foot and leg were working, I was walking, and I was "on my own" again.

My speech therapists at the new hospital were very sweet and gave me a lot of personal attention, but I wasn't making much progress in that area either. They were trying but just didn't have enough experience with my triple-edged sword of dysarthria (difficulty in speech production, specifically with sequencing and forming words), apraxia (knowing exactly what I want to say but a disruption in the part of the brain that sends the signal to the tongue muscle to say the word makes it difficult) and aphasia (neural pathways for language comprehension were damaged or destroyed). So, the time I spent with three different alternating therapists was not productive. With all our therapy slowdowns, and the length of time that had passed since my stroke and hospitalization, we decided to take a break and consider other locations and therapies that were available in an expanded area.

CHAPTER *Nine*

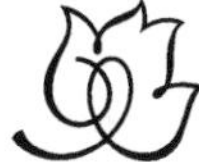

In the meantime, we decided I should take Brandon and go to visit my parents for some rest and relaxation. On June 2ND, Momma flew here so she could accompany us on a return flight to my hometown the next day. I was really nervous about flying, about leaving the security of the known, vs. facing the unknown, about everything! The flight was uneventful except Brandon kept wanting to get down and roll on the floor, but that kept my mind off everything else.

Then, just about the time we started our descent, I had a pain in the back of my head like I used to get every time I flew when I was younger. Then it wasn't terrifying – now it was! Momma was about to ring the stewardess and tell her to have EMS meet us when we landed, but as quickly as it began, it was over. Very scary – if it hadn't already happened to me most of my life, I would have been hysterical. Daddy was waiting at the bottom of the escalator with a big smile and big open arms. Brandon was extremely happy to see him ...and most especially to be off the plane.

The drive to the house was troubling - I didn't know if I would remember anything or everything. As we turned into the cul-de-sac, it all came flooding back. *Oh yes ...I could remember it all! This snippet of information proves that retained memories that aren't lost is dependent upon which hemisphere of the brain they were stored in prior to a stroke.*

The entire visit was wonderful. I had Momma make a list of every restaurant I loved, and she would order food for take-out, so I could enjoy it at home without having to get out. Brandon had a great time, swimming every day and playing with his Auntie Ann and J.J. who took him shopping and to the zoo. My Aunt Victoria came to town to visit too, and she and Ann and Momma even took him to Lakeside Amusement Park to ride the rides. My friend Kim came to visit me and brought several orders of Rollo's Tacos (an area natives' favorite) -- we ate and laughed and had a great time. Maurine, another friend, came over and brought me up to speed on her colorful life. All of Momma's friends came to see me and told me how good they thought I was doing. I had an appointment with my lifelong favorite hairstylist and got my hair cut short so I could manage it better. This made me feel pretty and gave me a "new outlook on life."

Every day I would get up and drive to Pinewoods Park for a walk. It took me quite a bit longer to walk each lap than it used to take for me to run it when I was training, but I felt like I was doing myself good. It was much easier for me to just sit on the sofa and do nothing, but that didn't do anything toward building my self-esteem. On my fourth outing, I realized that my brace was rubbing a large blister on my heel and this was something I knew I had to watch out for. Since I had no direct feeling in that foot it could have been dangerous because a deep sore is hard to heal, and I would be forced to quit walking ...something I didn't want to do.

It seemed just about the time we were getting comfortable, and in a "fun groove", it was time to go back home to Jaime and Snowman. I wasn't nearly as nervous about the return flight, and since it was late in the afternoon Brandon slept most of the way home. What an excellent summer "therapy trip".

CHAPTER *Ten*

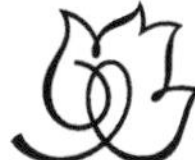

Since everything going on in my training program had basically stalled, my parents began wondering about getting me back to the "tried and true" ITLRT program. On one of the last therapy appointments at the hospital I was presently going to, Daddy was walking in to sit in on my speech therapy session. He passed a young woman in the gym who was wearing a new technology electronic leg stimulating unit (ELSU) and was walking without any appearance of a limp. Before he went into speech with me, he went back to Momma and told her to watch for the young woman to see how well she was walking.

Momma went in search of the woman and watched her throughout her therapy. As she was leaving the gym, Momma introduced herself and asked if she might have a moment of her time. The woman replied, "Of Course." Their conversation lasted the hour that I was in therapy, and when I came out, Stacye introduced herself to me. We found out she had exactly the same type of dissected artery stroke that I had suffered, but hers had been 7 years before mine. Her mother was a whiz at computer research and had also found the ELSU that she had been using for four years. More importantly, she highly recommended an occupational therapist who was independent of hospitals and who made house visits. Momma got her name and made up her mind that this was the approach we needed to take towards a better tomorrow for me.

She called Belinda, had her meet us at a soda shop that week, and a deal was struck. Belinda came to my house the following week and we started our therapy relationship in October. It was exciting to get back into a routine where I felt like I was making progress again and where a therapist was trying new things to make me push myself. It gave me incentive to do exercises and strength building that I had been hesitant to do before.

With Halloween approaching, I asked Jaime to get in the attic and hand me the boxes of decorations stored there. It took me a couple of days, but I decorated the house with all the goodies that I had always displayed before. When Momma and Daddy came to pick up Brandon to take him to Sea World, they were quite surprised and happy to see that I had been able to put everything out. Belinda said she had never seen a house decorated like mine (lots and lots of decorations saved from several years of fixing up classrooms and diagnostic offices), and she was very impressed with the way things looked and what I was able to accomplish.

In planning ahead, Momma had contacted Georgia by e-mail to see if she would be interested in coming back to work with me. After checking with Dr. McCall, and making sure we had severed our ties with the other associated hospital, my friend and speech therapist extraordinaire returned to help me in November 2010. It was only a few sessions until I was making good progress in my speech activities again.

It wasn't long before the holiday season was upon us. That year, with Jaime's help getting the things out of the attic, I had the house totally decorated before my parents' monthly visit the first week of December. When I say decorated, I mean each room in the house had a display of some sort of beautiful antique figurines, musical ornaments, carved candlesticks with wreaths, and all types of handmade decorations passed down through generations. Jamie also put up lights on the exterior eaves of the house, no small feat since our house has roof lines that are 25 feet tall in some places. Momma brought some more outside lights and ornaments, so we finished up everything that week. I just love Christmas and all the pretty lights; it is a very special time in the Thomas household – and I was thrilled that I had been able to do the decorating myself before my parents arrived. Since all my siblings, my niece and nephews, and my aunt were planning to visit my hometown for Christmas, Momma flew in to be with us on December 20th and was here to enjoy playing in the snow with Brandon (me too,) and taking him to see the lights around the neighborhood. I think 2010 will be the first Christmas he remembers when he is older.

We got up early Christmas morning and watched our special little guy enjoy Santa's gifts. It had been a labor of love to purchase things I thought he wanted and to get them wrapped and under the tree. Momma cooked a delicious Holiday dinner which we enjoyed early in the afternoon so she could get to the airport and catch a 3 p.m. flight home; she got there in time to spend Christmas evening with the rest of the family. I left the decorations up for a couple of days but took them down before New Year's Day. I remember Mammy's warning that it was bad luck to take things out of the house on the first day of the year, so I like to get it done early.

CHAPTER
Eleven

2011 – The New Year always offers an opportunity to make changes for the better, and that's why folks make resolutions that they hope to keep. I am looking forward to more progress in all my therapies. Too many times the past couple of years I've asked God "Why me?" Now I found myself praying for His help and guidance in gaining more strength and being able to communicate better in 2011. Speaking clearly would be my number one answered prayer.

Momma and Daddy made another trip back the first week of February for Brandon's fourth birthday party. We made party reservations at Party-! -Party-! -Party! for Brandon and six little friends to enjoy his special day with him. Ann, Leigh, Kay, Ryan and Victoria all drove in and stayed with my parents at the Hilton Garden Inn. That gave Brandon a place to "camp out" overnight and swim for two days. Brandon had a funny child's impression of the hotel – when Daddy and Momma took him back after the party, so he could swim again, he said, "Oh, we're going back to the Museum." Ann said maybe he thought it was a place for old stuff since many of the guests that were there that weekend were attending a reunion and they were very old ...that plus the fact that all the walls in the lobby were covered with large pictures. At any rate, that gave all of us a big chuckle. Everybody enjoyed watching him celebrate a birthday that seemed to come too soon *...our baby is growing up and certainly doesn't like it when his Mama and Mimi call him "Baby".*

I continued to make progress and gain more confidence in myself and my driving. On March 12th, I could cross my right leg over the left one. Another big "PLUS" for me is being able to tie my tennis shoe laces with one hand. My sister Ann is in awe of this ability and keeps practicing and trying to do it herself. So far ...no cigar! Every accomplishment, even something like that, is recorded as a major milestone for me. Also, I started taking Brandon to day school; first time was on March 14TH. It was good to see the women in the office and to meet his new teachers. They seemed happy to see me again, and I was sure delighted to be there.

Daddy had been communicating via e-mail with my Aunt Sue for two or three months, and she had invited us to come to her ranch for a visit. So, on April 19TH Daddy and Momma drove down to pick Brandon and me up, and we all traveled to see Aunt Sue and Uncle Howard. It was good for my "heart" to be back in touch with her again. Brandon loved being at their place in the country, most especially running around the property, and messing with their three donkeys. Really tame and loved to be petted, but we didn't ever open the gate and get in the pasture with them. We decided to save that for another trip. Since that was a reunion of sorts and we really didn't know how things were going to go, we only stayed over one night and then returned home late the next day, which was Friday before Easter

Aunt Sue asked if I wanted the two white rocking chairs that had been on Granny and Granddad's back porch and I was very excited about that. They will look so good on our patio and give people a comfortable place to sit. Momma and Daddy got up very early Sunday morning and hid all of Brandon's eggs; so, when he got up and found everything, he immediately had a chocolate overload from gobbling up Russell Stover candy eggs. It was a good thing we got an early start because it turned cold and started raining at about one o'clock.

Daddy and Momma had planned to head west the next morning, but I talked them into staying one more day so Daddy could watch my therapy with Belinda. The big news, and the highlight of that visit, was a surprise I had for Momma. Since she had been working with my arm, I was able to pull it up and around behind Momma and give her a big two-armed hug. We were both so happy we cried. Time spent with my family is great therapy in itself for me.

One of the things I have always enjoyed doing is working in the yard, so as soon as the days started getting sunshiny and warm, it was back outside for me. It took about two weeks, but I managed to get all the dead undergrowth and weeds pulled out of the flower beds around the house. I always feel so "renewed" when things are cleaned out and ready for the new plants of summer. Also, on Daddy's last visit he went to a nursery with me and we picked out some evergreen bushes, a silver leaf maple tree and a couple of japonicas to plant in the back yard …so I've kept an eye on them to report on their growth progress. He always grumbled about the soil here being "Southern Fried Gumbo" but he loved getting out there and digging and helping me.

Whenever I start feeling remorseful about not making the progress I think I should, I realize what a blessing it is that I'm able to go out in the yard and get the gardening done. If I could just accomplish as much with my speaking, I would be overjoyed.

Since I have started getting out more and shopping at the mall vs. on-line, I have found that I am not able to explain myself to clerks, the old gentleman who assists females pumping gas at the station, doctor's receptionists, etc. Momma is aware of this, so we have both decided I should have a little laminated card to hand to people instead of trying to communicate unsuccessfully. I'm just sorry we didn't do this before because it works like a charm. It has a short explanation that I've had a stroke and cannot converse fluently, and assistance will be appreciated; all my personal information is listed, plus Brandon's name and address, Jaime and Momma's names, addresses and telephone numbers. Now I no longer have the fear that I'm going to get somewhere and not be able to tell anybody anything, especially in an emergency.

Brandon's and my summer trip home was scheduled for June 21ST. Just to get in practice for swimming I decided he and I could go to the Crest Pool near our house. We had a great time …made him happy to get out with me. The next day, I took him to the Club Road Pool because not as many teenagers go there. Momma came down and stayed for a couple of days and then we all traveled back together. I really enjoyed being at home sunning by the pool and exercising in the water, getting massages, eating good Mexican food and being "spoiled." Oh Boy! The weeks passed too quickly and on July 24TH we all made the Eastward Ho! trip home. Momma just stayed a couple of days before leaving again and she and Brandon cried all the way to the airport. She told him he could come see her all by himself, so on August 13TH she and Daddy drove back down here again and took him home with them for a ten day stay. He really enjoyed being the center of attention and doing all the things Mimi and Granddad do with him. He just didn't like the 10-hour ride back and sat in his car seat with a blanket over his head for most of the trip. Four days later, it was off to Log Cabin Lodge; on the first day of school I made it a point to take him by myself. As prearranged - none of us like goodbyes - my parents left while I was gone so it was an emotional day for me.

Another milestone day on September 7TH. I shaved *both* my legs for the first time and by being a contortionist was also able to finally shave under my left arm. I'm happy to add this to my "I CAN DO IT LIST" of major accomplishments! People don't realize what they take for granted on a daily basis, and good personal grooming is something very important for my self-esteem!

It seemed like the month went by in a flash. I got ambitious and asked Jaime to help me get the Halloween decorations out of the attic so I could put them up early ...very early, so everything inside and outside of the house was up by the fourth week of September when Momma arrived.

On September 28TH, I had my first "girls' night out" since my stroke. It was a fun, memorable evening with my friends, Christy and Shawna. Instead of going any place fancy, we chose a comfortable restaurant called Consuelo's Mexican Food; for me, it felt like the neatest place ever …free like a bird for the evening.

On my birthday the next Monday, Momma made my favorite strawberry cake and cooked meat enchiladas. Of course, I ate too much, so I felt rotten the next day because I wasn't used to that kind of food.

On Thursday, we went to Northeastern Campus for speech therapy, then stopped to do a little shopping. On the way home, Momma talked me into joining her to get a flu shot. Afterward, we went home, and I stretched out for a nap, so Momma went to her room to read and she fell asleep. About 4:30 she woke up and was getting ready to pick up Brandon when she noticed her shoulder was sore where she got the shot. She came in and woke me up and asked if I felt okay. I said "No, I hurt all over and I'm hot." She felt my forehead and told me I was running a temperature. After picking our boy up, she checked on me again and I was burning up with fever. There are so many pain killers I can't take that she just gave me some Tylenol and kept cold compresses on my head and neck. She called Daddy and told him to Google reactions to flu vaccinations. I had *all* of them. The next day I was still running a temp of 100 so he called their doctor and asked him about it. The doctor said that if a person has that kind of reaction, it generally means that their immune system is compromised and *without* the shot *if* I had contracted the flu, I would have wound up very ill and in the hospital. “Thanks Momma,” I thought.

More changes were in the wind. At the suggestion of Georgia, my great speech therapist, I began seeing a new occupational therapist at Northeastern. (she had been keeping track of me through the hospital patient portal and I was grateful for her help in referring me to her friend.) For reasons unknown to me, Belinda was slowly pulling back from coming to my house. Perhaps the long travel time or perhaps the agreed-upon price for each session didn’t make it worth her while. But, for whatever reason her visits had dwindled to about once every two weeks and that wasn’t sufficient. So, on October 19th, I had my first appointment with Karrie at Northeastern. She gave me some negative heel stretch exercises to do ...my legs really hurt so that let me know that my calves hadn’t been getting a proper workout! With change comes more change – Karrie didn’t like the Bionic device. Instead, she insisted that I wear an articulated hard brace again. I was a little upset because I thought I had seen the last of braces, but changes have always challenged me so I’m on a different tack now. Time will tell.

As a late birthday present Momma bought me tickets to fly home for an R&R visit, so on October 20th, I made the trip. I was a little apprehensive about dealing with security people at the airport, but Jaime was with me in case they asked something I couldn’t answer. Piece of cake! Only one hiccup – when the plane landed, we were twenty minutes early; I was in the first seat and got off in a hurry so when I got to the bottom of the elevator there was nobody there! Daddy and Momma were running in the front door about the time I got half-way down the entrance concourse and they were horrified and apologetic. I got a laugh in on them.

I had a therapy massage with Dolores every day and she really loosened up my arm and shoulder. Also, the magic hair colorist Malena turned me into a blond again! First time I've had highlights since January of 2009. Cut my hair in a "chic bob" - shorter in the back than the front sides - and I felt really "stylin." Also, I was really pleased with myself because I took a shower without the chair and shaved my legs while standing up on October 21ST– another "Hooray Day" for Kiirstin! (Since I had been continuing with my negative heel stretches in front of the fireplace, Daddy cut me a board to take back home in my luggage so I could continue doing them here.)

Of course, it was heavy, and the baggage handler asked me if I was carrying bricks in my suitcase. Home Again, Home Again on the 24th

Momma ordered a stand for my hair dryer so I could fix my hair by myself! As I've pointed out before, women use both hands to accomplish their personal grooming, so it is hard for anybody to imagine what it takes to get the job done using only one! Having to hold the dryer in one hand, putting it down and brushing a tress up, letting the brush go to pick up the dryer – repeatedly – and not being successful half the time is more than frustrating. So, the first time I tried the new stand that holds the dryer securely to the countertop and all I had to do was brush and curl the locks of hair, **and it worked,** I was extremely happy. The next day, November 9TH, I picked up a new articulated leg brace. I felt like everybody was looking at me but knew that I'd get used to it. That is another thing that stroke survivors must endure – and I'm sure people don't mean to be rude – but staring at you as you approach, looking at you like you're to be pitied or unattractive, is very disheartening.

Hoo-ray! I woke up on November 12TH and decided to drive through our favorite donut shop's service line for the first time. Fun "first" times! Brandon went with me, but I couldn't remember how to say donut holes, so we just bought whole donuts.

When I decided it was time to get the Christmas decorations out and the lights put up on the house before Thanksgiving, Jaime wasn't even surprised. In fact, we had fun getting things down and placed outside. I was so *very thankful* that this joyful job was something I could accomplish by myself.

For the first time, we decided to spend Christmas Eve and Christmas Day alone at home ...just the three of us. Nice quiet family time together and Brandon was excited that Santa Claus brought "toys". Two days later, for the first time he and I flew to Daddy's and Momma's house by ourselves! As usual, Brandon was happy to get off the plane and even happier to get to Daddy and Momma's house. All the Christmas decorations were still out, and we had presents under the tree just like Christmas Day. Ann, J.J., Leigh, Scott, Kay, and Aunt Victoria came over and we all had a wonderful holiday visit together for the first time in a couple of years. During our little *winter vacation,* we went to the park several times even though it was cold. Daddy and I walked around the park together - the distance is one mile, so it was a real workout for me – and Momma watched Brandon ride his new bicycle on long stretches of the empty parking lot without worrying about cars.

When we were ready to start the trip home, we knew there was some bad weather at the state line that we were going to have to navigate through. It was *less than wonderful* because the drive time is normally 10 hours, but we spent 8 hours maneuvering through terrible ice, sleet and snow, which resulted in taking 14 nail-biting hours to get there. On the Interstate with an 80-mph speed limit, we drove no more than 40 mph at any time. Lots of wrecks so we had to creep along behind semi-trucks to be able to stay in the tire tracks they had plowed through. Not nice ...don't want to do that again anytime soon. However, once again, Brandon was a good little traveler and my leg only got uncomfortable the last hour of the trip.

I was anxious to get the Christmas decorations and tree stored for another year, so as I packed everything in boxes and storage tubs, Momma and Daddy helped me put them back in the attic

Time to get back to normal and welcome the new year

Moving Forward. *This portion of my personal journey down an unexpected and untraveled road is a compilation of recollections, accomplishments and victories in the years that include my hard-fought partial recovery. I have a plaque on my bedroom wall that reads "You Have a Road to Walk as You Go Through Life That Is Yours Alone – You May Have Others That Go With You But They*

Cannot Walk In Your Stead". I have had more than several loved ones walk beside me, but the completion of my journey has been up to me and my God. He alone knows where and how it will end.

2012 Another New Year! I have mentally reviewed everything that transpired the past year and I'm thankful. I have only one regret - that is the fact that I'm still so challenged with my ability to speak. Aphasia and Apraxia are two inconceivable disabilities to deal with.

I'm still attending speech therapy sessions at the Conversational Learning Center twice a week. As I explain over and over to the therapists assigned to work with me, I can picture the word in my mind, but when I try to physically pronounce it, my tongue and muscles just don't work. Other times, I remember the word but can't picture it in my mind. Just makes me want to scream! Sometimes I need to repeat in my head what people are saying several times in order to understand them. This, of course, causes them to think there is a disconnect, so they try to "help me" say the word I'm struggling with, which causes a further delay in my thought process. Additionally, I've come to realize that any background noise is extremely aggravating to me – I must utilize all my concentration on what I'm trying to learn or what people are saying. Visual imprinting is important - when reading learning materials, using highlighters to imprint the words in my brain is very helpful. One of these days, somebody is going to invent an audio/visual machine much like the virtual ones being used by scientists, and those of us who have suffered brain injuries are going to be able to plug into video, put on earphones and talk like magic. *I just wish I could be the one to invent that magic carpet ride.*

In January Momma and I went to the learning center for a couple of sessions, and to Northeastern for a follow-up with Karrie. She stresses that I must adjust my gait to take exaggerated steps lifting my knees up and down (like marching), and then roll my step-down heel first and finish on my toe. Unless I practice walking that way I am doomed to swing my leg out and drag my toe on the follow-through. I walked a couple of times doing that and it makes a difference in my toe drag. More practice needed to accomplish this change.

While Momma and I were taking care of all the things on my "To Do List," we went to Savers Club and applied for a credit card in my name so I can buy gasoline at the location near my house. I can also buy groceries and things in the store. While we were there we did a "test run" to make sure the card worked. I went back by myself on the 17TH of February and then again on the 28TH and could pump my own gas. Yea! More independence for Kiir!! I really don't give myself enough credit because I think I'm not progressing fast enough but everybody tells me I'm able to do a lot that other catastrophic stroke victims can't even think about doing. As a matter of fact, when I mentioned this concern to my physical therapist she told me to celebrate my baby steps. So, now I'm going to always remember Tuesday, March 6, 2011, the first time I went to Brook's, picked up everything we needed for the house, went through checkout, got my groceries to the car, and unpacked everything when I got home. I accomplished everything I needed to do *by myself* and that made me feel very good. Thank You, God.

Some time ago I told Momma I didn't want the maid service to come back because I could do a much better job than any outside help. Also, the exercise helps me with my strength and flexibility. On March 10TH, I gave the house a good cleaning in preparation for my parents' coming to visit the following week. They planned to only be here for a couple of days, but it was important to me for the house to look good for them. They were very impressed with the way the house looked and how good it smelled! Totally spic-and-span with scented candles burning in every room – I was proud of myself, to say the least. Momma says I can just call myself "My Pretty Maid" (the name of the first recital dance I performed when I was 3 years old) and that she will happily pay me to clean the house, which will give me pocket money that is "just for me." *My Pretty Maid Cleaning Service* gives me a paycheck every month and adds to my growing sense of independence and accomplishment.

Momma came back on April 1ST and stayed almost two weeks ...I really look forward to her visits, so we can go shopping, and this time we bought a new light fixture for the kitchen ceiling, one for the guest bath, and another for the master bath. Then, we knew we'd have to "surprise" Daddy and tell him he has to come back down here to install them.

We signed Brandon up for T-Ball Baseball Camp. He seems to really like it so perhaps this is a sport we can all be involved in through his school years. I'm a T-ball mom so I've ordered a team shirt with his number on it. Love It! He is in a group of little boys who have either played one year or this is their first time out, so it is fun to watch them trying to follow instructions. Unfortunately,

Brandon and his friend Landon have more fun throwing dirt clods in the air and trying to catch them with their gloves than they spend time catching baseballs.

As the end of the season approached, Brandon's team started being on the winning side rather than the bottom. When we found out they were going to be in the playoffs we let Momma and Daddy know so they made a trip down to watch them play. Got clear to the "world series" and only lost the next-to-the-last game. And I absolutely *loved* being a team Mom, wearing a red shirt with his number on the back outlined in rhinestones. Too much fun for everyone!!

It hardly seems possible that my "baby" is leaving the private school he has attended since he was 18 months old. Time has absolutely flown by. A graduation ceremony, complete with caps and gowns, was attended by all parents and grandparents. At the end of the ceremony the students all stood and said aloud what they want to be when they grow up. Some said policemen, teachers, soldiers and doctors, but Brandon said, "I'm going to be a Fireman." Since he has always been so enthralled with fire trucks and ambulances, and tells various adults that "those men" come when you need help, maybe this might really be what he wants to do. I just want him to be happy in his work and am looking forward to seeing what road my boy travels as he grows to be a man. I thank God, every day for sparing me and giving me the opportunity to be a part of this growing up process. It certainly could have turned out differently.

On my grandmother's birthday (July 15TH) my son got his first stitches. I had a bad headache and stayed in bed to try to let it pass; Brandon was with Jaime who was watching TV. He heard a big crash in the kitchen and went running in to find a chair turned over and Brandon on the floor crying. Apparently, he had decided to get in the cabinet to get some candy in one of the upper shelves and his foot slipped, and down he went, hitting his chin on the way down. It bled quite a bit and we thought the gash looked like it needed stitches, so we paid a visit to the emergency room (his first). To say that he didn't want any kind of a shot to deaden his chin for the required stitches *is putting it mildly*. He just kept yelling "No needles, no needles" repeatedly so the doctor said they would make two small stitches without any pain killer. Absolute madness. It was over very quickly, and he acted like it wasn't too bad. Brandon scares me from that standpoint – his pain threshold is extremely high and he is quite fearless (except for needles, that is). I took pictures of his little chin and swollen upper lip and sent it to his grandparents, so they could worry along with me. A "red letter day" for my little tough guy.

In late August, Brandon started school at Hillside Elementary about four blocks from the house. It has certainly been interesting so far. Momma said she thinks the teachers at day school mainly tried to keep the kids from hurting each other vs. teaching them much of anything. This is *not* the case now, so I'm trying to get his attitude adjusted towards listening, listening, listening, and being quiet. However, he's only five years old, so the attitude adjustment continues and will for some time.

Daddy and Momma came to Dallas to celebrate my birthday – and to install all the light fixtures we purchased earlier in the year. Also, they made it a point to go to speech therapy with me so they could see how well I've been doing. I'm still working on my problem with aphasia, but I can sense a breakthrough might be right down the road. Reading aloud to myself is an exercise that my speech therapist insists will help me get there. She made arrangements for me to receive a "book reader" through the state, whereby I can listen to books and practice reading aloud as I'm listening ...then during the next therapy session, we talk about what I've listened to/learned. This helps with my cognition and also lets them know my progress in understanding oral cues.

2013 - I found out about a site on-line called Lumosity that has exercises to help with brain function and reading. When I told Daddy about it he checked out the exercises, took a couple of the sample tests and thought it would probably help, so he bought a subscription for a year to see how I like it. So far, so good, my first score is 171 so I've got lots of room to improve.

Another checkmark in the box for me being independent ...I ordered some new tennis shoes on-line vs. the expensive brand that we previously bought here. They look and feel good. Having to order two different sizes was a challenge, but the company I found advertised on the web specializes in shoes for people like me who need unmatched sizes, so it was a success! Yea, Kiir!!

Brandon is still having some behavior issues in school but the "Code Red" daily reports are fewer. This, of course, necessitates my visiting the school and consulting with his teachers. Through all of this I can't seem to help him understand the importance of applying himself and doing the very best he can. I try to remember my own feelings about school and my bad behavior when I recorded spelling words on the teacher's tape recorder, accidently killed the fish by overfeeding them, hid in the locker room instead of getting on the school bus to go home, and forging the check to buy books; each of these actions infinitely more serious than him not turning in homework. I try not to think about my screaming and door slamming at that age, but I imagine more sinister reasons for him doing it based it on my lasting impairment from the stroke. Being a psychologist should help me work through these rough spots in the road, but I am unable to do so because I feel I am failing him. I've just got to work on my own self-esteem, but that is hard to do because inside I feel I'm damaged.

Almost before I knew the year was flashing by, the Holidays arrived. Early in December I decided it was time to start getting the house decorated for Mammy's favorite time of the year. Her love of all things Christmas - the decorations, lights, food, hospitality, and traditions associated with this lovely holiday - is something she passed on to my mother, and my mother to me. It is a time of year when I remember her with so much love and miss being with her. I decided to make a double batch of Mammy's canasta mix and peppermint bark, so I could package it up and share with Victoria, Cody, and Momma and Daddy. I was delighted that I was able to fix those things by myself and get them wrapped, delivered to the post office, and mailed. Once again, baby steps enabling me to do memorable things. Momma and Daddy drove down here on the 26th to celebrate a late Christmas with us. There was snow on the ground and it was very cold, so we didn't do much except stay inside and visit. DeWitt and Anna had the family over on the 27th and included Momma and Daddy. That was a nice opportunity for everybody to be together. Really a nice evening with everyone.

Every one of these opportunities to be with loved ones has taken on a new meaning for me the last four years. The love of family is an important part of my life.

I had an occupational therapy session scheduled at Northeastern on the 29TH so Daddy and Momma went with me. They liked my new OT Carolyn a lot. While talking with her, it was decided that we should purchase a therapy aid for my hand. It is a device that looks like the bottom half of a glove that my hand fits into, and with the use Velcro straps and springs it helps me grasp and pick up small items. Object of this is to enable me to pick up a ball, or pen, or eating utensil and move it from one place to another and put it down. Good for picking up clothes or shoes, or setting the table. I'm looking forward to receiving it.

Another thought from the past and things resulting from those actions: I've over-looked writing about the fact that in February of 2011, almost 2 years after my stroke Daddy was researching stroke therapy devices online and found one that was supposed to assist patients in regaining strength and dexterity in their affected arms. Nothing would make him happy until Momma ordered one. That was the easy part, because none of the hospitals that I had gone to had trained therapists who could assist me in utilizing the machine which is called UMYOM. It is battery powered and when sensors are taped to the arm muscle to be used, the machine delivers a shock that causes the muscle to contract, thereby assisting the patient in raising/extending their arm. The therapist that I had coming to the house didn't much want to work with it, preferring to get me to do strength training and repetitious movements. We actively searched for medical centers in the area to find a trained therapist who is willing to give it a try.

Finally, in June of 2012, I received an out-of-the-blue invitation from *UMYOM* stating that there would be a "get acquainted" reception at local convention hotel ...only thing wrong with that was it was right in the middle of the time I was going to be at my parents' house for our annual summer visit. I kept the information, and in September, Momma called the people and asked them if they had hired anyone in my area who was actively using the E-STIM device. They said they had an OT at a nearby hospital who was conducting trials. She was very cautious when setting up my first appointment to see if they could help. Because of my not being under their insurance umbrella their therapy fees would not be covered; so, I put my name on a call list to let me know when my insurance provider applied to be included in their roster of approved insurances.

In September of 2013 we received a call from the hospital we contacted, and they said that beginning in the new calendar year (2014) my insurance coverage would be in effect for outpatient treatment. On January 8, I made an appointment to see the OT (who had been there working all along – what a waste of valuable time from my standpoint). She was very dedicated, very experienced, and very knowledgeable. We had adequate time with her to fully acquaint myself with the unit. When the UMYOM unit quit working, she took the initiative to return it to the manufacturer to have it repaired and the software upgraded.

2014 is gonna' be keen! Might as well have a rhyming motto ...there's lots to do this year ...lots of giant steps I'd like to take. I've got an embroidered plaque on my "positive thoughts wall" that Mother made for me that reads "She's Not Where She Was Before ~ She's Not Where She Is Going ~ But She's On Her Way." That is going to be my mantra for 2014!

We got the UMYOM unit back on the 18TH of February and are finally working with it after almost three years. On the plus side, I've physically progressed during those three years by getting stronger and becoming surer of my own physical abilities. *And*, this therapist is not anti-ELSU like previous ones have been. Because of all the changes I've worked through, I've certainly learned that therapists have definite ideas (and dislikes) about methods of therapy that they personally have not used, but I'm sure they feel like it's for good reason. Most importantly, they have experienced different degrees of success with their patients. Because of this, various methods/ trials/theories have all been a **part of my road traveled** in attempting to regain the use of my arm and leg. Thinking positively – which is of utmost importance to me and my psyche - without these experiences, I would have just been someplace sitting around without the benefit of *somebody trying to the best of their ability* to help me, so I'm very grateful for that. I'm glad my attitude is still that I'm never going to give up.

Also, my own determination to overcome the physical limitations caused by the stroke has been enhanced by two recurring things: (1) My father's continued search for cutting-edge devices that are not mainstream or widely used, and his desire that they be acquired, and (2) my mother's ability to figure out ways to buy the devices for me. As I have always known, their unwavering belief that I will do everything to excel and overcome obstacles I face is what encourages me to go forward. That, plus believing in myself, and the love I have for my son, makes me think I can move mountains!

On February 18TH, I had another "Red Letter Day" - my hand exerciser was put to good use. I was able to pick up a small rubber ball 15 times, squeeze it and throw it down. Hoo-Ray! Won't be too long before I can pick up something smaller like a pencil or a pen. Heck! Think big!! Let's go for a bowling ball.

What better way to start off the month of March than to take a milestone step towards ...forever? I finally can get in my shower, wash my hair and shave my legs all without having to sit on my safety chair. Little steps equal giant leaps in my progress and that equals *kudos* for Kiirstin!

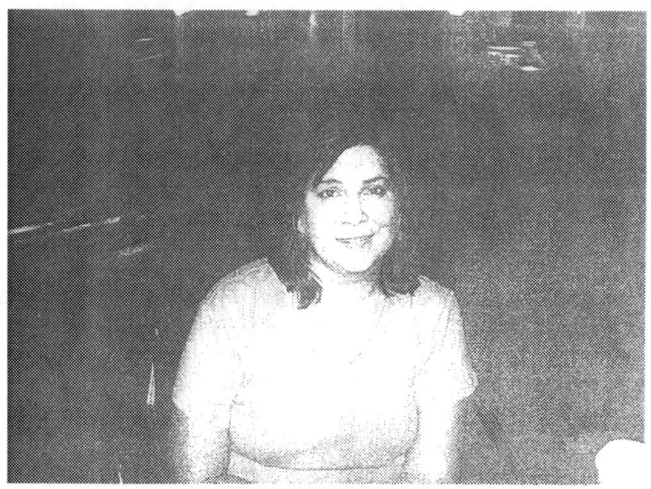

Kiirstin

Momma came in for her regular visit and I had plans for her that I knew would be exciting for both of us. I had been wanting to visit a good friend from my special education teaching days. She lives out in the country and it is a 50-mile round trip from my house to get there. Momma called her and made plans to bring lunch and drive out to see her and her new baby daughter. (I didn't tell Momma that I hadn't driven out there since a year before my stroke, or that it involves miles and miles of driving on back roads through small towns.) As we were driving around she wasn't very optimistic that I knew where we were going. For just a few minutes, I was a little concerned that maybe I had made a wrong turn. However, I just had to make one U-turn to go back to find the right driveway, *but I did it!* Absolutely an exhilarating feeling to accomplish something like that. Makes me so happy I could almost cry, because in the back of my mind I know what I'm doing, but there is always a niggling doubt. Nice visit, nice day.

Daddy and Momma drove down for a visit the first week in May (coinciding with Mother's Day). Of course, they came to visit, but there were two things of importance in Daddy's mind - to help me finish planting both the front and back yards with grass sod and to go see Brandon play baseball. Luckily, his team won 2 games (they lost two, both against the first and second place teams), and he was happy to have Granddad and Mimi there to cheer him on. He sure can hit the ball, and is almost the fastest runner so he likes to get out there and try. As it turned out at the end of their season, due to a process of elimination and some good luck, Brandon's team won the trophy!

Brandon's 2nd grade year finished on a positive note. His teacher reported that he had made good progress and the only suggestion she had was for him to read, read, and read all summer. Since that was what I loved to do the most when I was young, my sister Ann and I read a lot together - or I would be quiet and just listen, I'm hoping Brandon will eventually find out how enjoyable it is to lose yourself in a good book. When that happens, he will learn to love reading. Right now, there is only one thing that interferes with that - his infatuation with video games. Taking away the screens is my best method of discipline ...about the only one that he pays attention to. When it comes time to read or go swimming, my best trading chip is "read first, and then you can." Moving forward ...3rd Grade ...hope he likes it

I received an invitation to attend a Retirement Dinner for a wonderful friend who was principal at a school where I once taught. I had serious misgivings about getting dressed up and going by myself and meeting all the people I knew were going to be there. I told Momma I didn't feel comfortable about going, but she insisted that it would be very good for me to go and interface with everybody and let them see how much I've improved, and how much I've been able to accomplish since they last heard about my stroke and the severity of my condition. I thought and thought and finally decided that I had everything to gain and nothing to lose by going, so I RSVP'd that I would be there. Worry, worry, worry, think, think, think ...it was great! I saw lots of people, many that I really liked, and, some that I remembered that I didn't like at all. I hadn't really thought about those individuals for these past few years, but in being with them again, the old feelings came flooding back. Our minds don't lose anything – they just put them on a back burner.

When debilitating times of despair periodically set in I'm especially disheartened over the fact that my professional career is undeniably over. I was extremely happy with the positive influence I was having with my special needs students and the progress they were making. I was making a measurable difference in their lives which was very exciting for them and rewarding for me. For a couple of years after my stroke, I had been hoping that I would overcome my apraxia and aphasia so that I might be able to return to work; perhaps in the areas of administering tests or possibly analyzing and diagnosing students after reading evaluations written by special education teachers. However, communication is key, and I have not yet mastered rudimentary conversation. I'll just have to keep trying and look to God for help.

Additionally, on the plus side of being employed, I appreciated being paid a salary well beyond what I had ever envisioned, and thus was an equal breadwinner for my family. The future looked bright and finances were not going to be a problem. Then, it all disappeared in a heartbeat. I have numerous feelings of inadequacy because of things associated with my stroke, but at the top of the list is the problem Brandon is having in school because I cannot be more interactive with his teachers; I fault myself for not being the social companion that my husband needs to advance in his job; I'm disappointed in myself for my inability to be an attractive, happy, loving wife and mother; I'm disappointed that the monetary impact my not being able to work has had on the family; the list goes on and on until I can reason with the woman inside of me and accept the fact that these feelings are not mine to bear alone, and are things I can do absolutely nothing about.

Our trip to Gulf Shores, Alabama, was very enjoyable this year. This time, my mother-in-law reserved a big beach house located directly on the shore where everybody could be together. Lots of hours of family time, playing in the sun, swimming in the Gulf, and eating good stuff. One of my challenges and/or victories that trip was the fact that the house had two flights of steep wood stairs. At first, I was nervous, but before we left I mastered getting up and down them with ease. It really is a blessing that Anna and DeWitt make this wonderful opportunity available for us to go enjoy a neat vacation that I'm sure Brandon will remember all his life.

Time has been flying by ...don't know if it is because my son is getting bigger, or I feel like I'm getting better, but

I get out and do more. It seems like every day I'm able to accomplish things that I thought were out of my reach, and then, happily, I find that I CAN do them. One of these milestones was on June 27TH; I decided that I could grasp a gallon of milk in my *right* hand (the one severely affected by the stroke) and carry it to the living room. *I did it!* What a wonderful "red letter day."

2015 - My main focus, as has been the case since I started at the communication/conversation/learning/ center, is primarily on my aphasia and apraxia. I'm compartmentalizing in my mind exactly what my physical limitations are that are keeping me from conversing. In part, *my* impatience with myself makes me frustrated, which just adds to the problem. This happens every day with well-meaning friends, my parents, and occasionally, professionals. When I reach a stumbling block trying to form a word I'm struggling with, they try to help me by guessing what I'm trying to say. Sometimes I say, "just a minute" but what I'm really thinking is "*shut up*" because interruptions in my thought process just push me back to square one and I must mentally start over again. Very difficult, to say the least, and I'm still struggling with this. I know I have a long road ahead of me, but I'm secure in the knowledge that I will achieve the goals I've set forth. May take more time than I had hoped, but it ***is*** going to happen. When I visit with my "bestest" friends who I've known forever, or some of my mother's friends who have watched me grow up and become who I am today, I am at ease with them and don't feel like I must say everything perfectly. When that is the case, vocalizing is effortless. When I am talking to Brandon about school, life in general, or expectations about his behavior, words come easily. Of course, Jaime and I know each other so well that there is no problem with our communication. It is only when I'm put in a position where I must respond to "on demand" questions that I freeze-up and must reply that I've had a stroke and need a moment before answering.

Jaclyn, my friend who oversees the communications lab program, offered me and my friend Staci the opportunity to volunteer at one of the Assisted Living Retirement Homes in the metropolitan area. She mentioned that several of the residents living there have speech impediments themselves, and many of them have difficulty walking and exercising. She said since Staci and I are both outgoing and have overcome problems caused by our strokes she thought we would be an inspiration to the people who hadn't been able to get past their impairments. Besides, she said she thought it would be beneficial for us to get out and be among the public and practice our communication skills that we had worked on so diligently. We accepted her suggested proposal and started "reporting for work" on Wednesdays and Fridays at 10 o'clock in the morning. It was heart lifting and made me feel like I was accomplishing a great deal. We visited with some of the folks but mainly helped set up the dining rooms for lunch by trimming fresh blossoms and arranging them in vases for the tables. We also double checked the place settings of dinner ware and silver-plate eating utensils and saw to it that napkins were folded correctly and placed properly. Little niceties like that were very much appreciated when the residents came in for meals. The old gentlemen seemed to walk straighter, the little ladies started wearing jewelry and combing their hair better, and conversation was more animated. It made me happy to be a part of something that made those folks who were somebody's grandparents feel a little more pampered those days I was working. Being there reminded me of my own grandparents and that made me feel like I was helping make the world a happier place for the residents who sometimes didn't have any visitors.

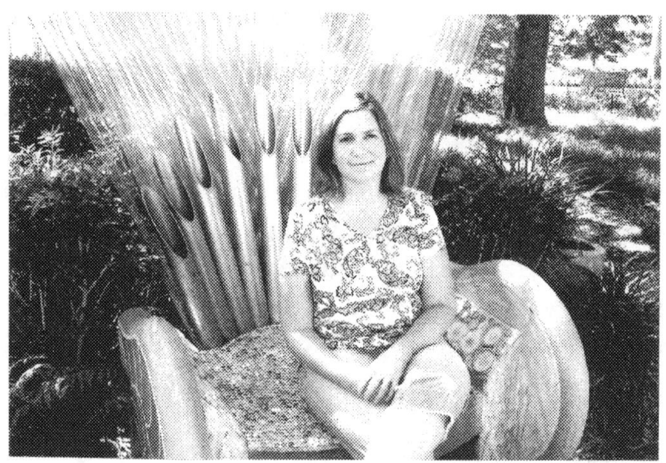

Kiirstin

2016 I am still finding that the on-line reading program is very valuable to me. Since I am a subscribing member, it keeps track of the progress I've made when taking tests. It is self-paced and there are categories that include vocabulary, cognition, math, problem solving and puzzles. It is encouraging to see that my first test score on an exercise I took 16 months ago was 171 and now my overall score as of February is 751. Just to see the increase in scores lets me know I'm improving every week and spurs me to work harder.

The area of the country where I live has been in the grip of a very severe drought for the last three years, and it is even more serious this year. There have been watering restrictions and no measurable rainfall, and as a result, all the grass in the front yard has dried up and died. When Momma was here in February, I talked to her about planting St Augustine but she said it wouldn't survive as long as there are freezing temperatures at night. Since she pooh-poohed the idea I didn't say anything further; but when the nights stayed warmer than the upper 40s I went to a local nursery to see if they had St Augustine for sale. They had just received new pallets of sod, so I bought 25 pieces that were 2ft x 4ft each. The men helped me by loading it into the trunk, but that was the easy part because *I had to UNLOAD it and PLANT it (lay it out flat with all sides touching so it wouldn't dry up)* when I got home. This is something that is extremely hard to do with two arms, but with me having only ***1 to use***, it was a huge mind-boggling accomplishment for me. Because I was determined this planting was going to live, I went out every afternoon, sat in a folding chair and sprinkled my new grass to give it the best chance to get a foothold and grow. When I called and told my parents what I had done, they were both absolutely amazed. Momma called me back the next day and told me she got off the phone and cried, because back in February she had made a mental note to call the nursery and arrange to have one of their subcontractors deliver and install the sod. She hadn't forgotten about the grass but decided it was still too early in the year ...but didn't tell me. She still couldn't believe I was able to do it alone and kept asking me over and over how I accomplished it. My answer was, I'm strong and I'm determined so I folded the sod pieces over and picked them up and carried them. I can say with certainty that nobody better get in an arm wrestling contest with me unless they are prepared to lose!

Point of Interest: Momma later told me she hadn't said anything more about planting the grass because she thought that might have encouraged me to move ahead by myself. She already knew what a huge job it was because she had installed 45 pieces of St Augustine sod right after my discharge from the hospital. She undertook that task after I first became aware the appearance of my front yard and complained bitterly about the dead grass. She hadn't planned her job well and didn't know there was nothing in the garage to use to move the 4-foot pieces from the car to the yard; so, she crisscrossed 3 pieces of sod at a time on the lid of our wheeled trash can and drug it back and forth 15 times. Must have been interesting to watch a crazy 68-year old woman doing that! She never mentioned a thing to me until the job was done, but said she called my Daddy every night while it was going on and told him she thought she was going to die in a pile of cow manure!

Prior to the beginning of the spring semester I contemplated not attending speech therapy sessions at the communications center lab. Although my being a clinical subject for incoming graduate students had been beneficial, after their initial assessments were in place, the outcome had been the same each year. They were learning by the experience, but I was not progressing. I felt as if I were taking up a slot that a more deserving patient might benefit from by participating. All things considered, I decided to discontinue attending the sessions even though I enjoyed the camaraderie and personal interaction with the other people. Perhaps if the class is re-structured to include a program involving a directed recovery protocol for Aphasia or Apraxia that would apply to an individual who has spent several years without much advancement, I would be a prime candidate. Until then, I've discontinued my speech therapy. In the meantime, I busy myself with attempting to assist my son in completing his math homework, accomplished by using methods I have no knowledge of. This almost falls under the same heading as my unsuccessful speech therapy. But each day brings new knowledge and determination, so who knows what is right around the corner?

Aunt Sue had been emailing me and talking about Brandon and me making another trip to the donkey "estate" for a visit (there are 3 of them and it is out in the country, so I've decided it must be an estate). We decided that July would be a good time to go see them and their beautiful property. For a little city boy, my son shows no fear about being around animals, and certainly isn't worried about driving golf carts or four wheelers. It made three people tired just to watch him and try to keep him from getting hurt and going back home with a battle scar. Another great visit with a favorite family member.

Our summer vacation this year was limited to a trip to my husband's sister's vacation home on the coast. We enjoyed the visitation with family members and Brandon's interaction with some older cousins. It gave me a chance to converse with adults in a familiar environment which is good exercise for me.

2017 has been a very eventful year and it is only August

In January, Momma and Daddy came in for an after-Christmas visit and to check on my car maintenance and road-worthiness. I mentioned that I would really like to start the year off right with a structured exercise program, so we visited a local fitness gym and talked to the manager about setting up a personalized program for me. We signed a contract for 3 sessions weekly for 6 months. I've seriously applied myself to the program and feel like I'm making good progress. Additionally, my personal trainer referred me to a doctor he is familiar with who has some success utilizing alternative medicine (acupuncture) to assist stroke survivors overcome spasticity in their limbs. I had my first appointment with him the end of the second week of my weight training, and since then have noticed a loosening of the tension in my arm. I feel like I'm taking steps to find a brand new me. At the very least I feel like a "jock" because I hurt all over. "No pain, no gain" as they like to say.

As April approached, my workout program and the acupuncture treatments were both going well, but after a particularly strenuous session, my left side began to hurt like something had been pulled. Following a couple of weeks of continued discomfort, I made an appointment to see my new OB/GYN to see what she thought about it. As with any new patient relationship she wanted x-rays, blood work, EKG's, etc. which I felt like were all routine. Imagine my surprise when her office called me to report that the x-rays showed a mass on my left ovary. It didn't take but two more appointments, and a contrast sonogram, for alarm bells to start ringing. A call to my Neurologist for his approval for the surgery – with a resultant CAT scan – paved the way for a complete hysterectomy. My previous OB/GYN had recommended that I have this same operation several years earlier because of a lifetime of ongoing female ailments. At that time, it was too soon after Brandon's birth and I wasn't ready to take that irreversible step, but here I was 8 years later, and the decision had been made for me. With a quick check to make sure Momma could fly down to provide tender loving care for both me and Brandon, final arrangements were made for me to have a robotic hysterectomy the 4TH of May.

Modern medicine is a marvelous thing. The use of medical robots in all types of surgery is fast becoming the norm. I, for one, had a very successful procedure that took an hour less time than usual; additionally, time spent in recovery and in my hospital room was limited to three days, and I came home with five one-inch incisions and a new lease on life.

My boy and I made our annual summer trek to my parents' house to (1) recharge my batteries and (2) give Brandon the opportunity to swim and exercise at his heart's content. Naturally, I got a lot of exercise in the pool and, as always, came back home with a nice healthy-looking tan. Being at my childhood home is always great, and when it's time to leave it seems to happen much too soon.

At this point in time, I watch in amazement at my son grows leaps and bounds. This is his first year attending Intermediate School (5TH grade). All the clothes I bought during the summer for the 2017/18 school year are too small! Some of them were exchanged for larger sizes but some of them were ordered on-line in June and cannot be returned. I've learned my lesson about buying end-of-school year bargains for the coming year because those items have now cost double. We have donated them to a children's store, so some little boy will get good use out of them.

The enjoyable on-line reading program has really helped me with my cognition, math knowledge and reading capability. I was very pleased when I took a "wrap up" quiz in September and my score was 1255. I looked back at my file when I began working problems and my very first score had been 171. This web site is an effective tool for keeping the brain challenged and working. And, I always live each day to the fullest and try my hardest, for a day not striving for my personal best is a day lost, and I keep hoping I will finally be able to converse fluently. Time and time again I am hampered when I face "on demand" speaking. If I practice what my responses will be in a particular situation I do very well. However, when a teacher, doctor, or somebody in a store asks me something off-the-cuff I know I have a "deer in the headlights" look on my face. So disturbing. The speech center, located in the parietal lobe of the left side of my head, is where all the damage occurred during the bleed when I had my stroke. This is the battle I'm fighting. I have read about, and understand, that I have the ability to visualize the word I want to say because my language recognition center is on the right side of my brain and it is undamaged. The motor aphasia and dysarthria on my left side are the culprits. Until some doctor or engineer invents a plug-in virtual device I can mortgage my soul to buy, or perhaps stem-cell experiments will identify someplace on my body where we can harvest "brilliant" cells to transplant in my head, I'll just have to keep on living my life as best I can, enjoying being with family and friends every day.

Any time I am experiencing feelings of inadequacy and then have to call up my inner voice of reason, I realize I'm very lucky to have experienced so many good things in life and have survived the unimaginable. For example, today, the smallest victory brings a smile to my face ...for the first time in eight years I *can feel mosquito bites* on my right leg ...I *can pull both arms up* and give people I love a hug around the waist I have a new carbon fiber brace and *can wear the same size shoe on both feet* ...little things mean a lot. And I Thank the Good Lord for His Blessings.

As unbelievable as it seems to me, another year is almost over. October is upon us and that means the end-of-year holidays aren't far behind. The older I get; the faster Brandon grows. It won't be long before he is a teenager and I'll be dealing with all the grief I used to cause my parents. Like the song goes, "the big wheel keeps on turning and the world spins 'round and 'round." Blessedly, our lives go on with hope for bright sunny days and starry nights.

Fortunately, perhaps out of self-preservation, after eight years I've progressed to the point that I'm no longer distressed with what people think about the way I look after my stroke. At first, I was terribly embarrassed about my limp, the fact that my arm doesn't hang correctly, and sometimes the corner or my mouth droops.

Now, I've arrived at a good place. I go shopping and I think I look good. I go to pick up Brandon at school and

I think I look good. I go to lunch with friends and I think I look good
I've got what I need.
Brandon cares for me
Jaime loves me.
I'm here to live my life another day with The Lord's Blessing

SPECIAL ACKNOWLEDGEMENTS

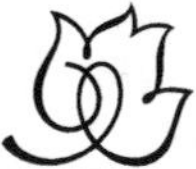

I would like to recognize and thank the people who have had such an impact on my life – and consequently played major roles in getting this book written. Without their medical expertise, assistance, guidance, love encouragement, and understanding, my return trip would have been much more difficult and not the positive and rewarding experience it has been.

My Husband	– My Love, Caregiver and Friend
My Son	– Who lights up my life
My Parents	– The most loving and supporting parents anyone could ever hope for
My Husband's Parents	– Dad^2 and Other Mother Always loving
My Brother and Two Sisters	– My cherished siblings

My Educator Peers and Friends at McArthur and Chanticleer Schools

The Neurologist who quickly recognized my dissected artery and saved my life

The Wonderful Qualified Neurologist who specializes in restoring hope and life

The Staffs at All Stroke Therapy Facilities who tried their best to help me heal

Lorene Glenn Rogers – Long time family friend whose caring insight, empathy and advice was a driving force behind getting this story written

ed States